Living
SMART

Living
SMART
LIFESTYLE CHANGE MADE SIMPLE

Joshua C. Klapow, Ph.D.

Clinical Psychologist, Associate Professor of Public Health,
University of Alabama at Birmingham, Alabama

Sheri D. Pruitt, Ph.D.

Clinical Psychologist and Behavioral Science Consultant

LIVING SMART
LIFESTYLE CHANGE MADE SIMPLE

iUniverse books may be ordered through booksellers or by contacting:

iUniverse
1663 Liberty Drive
Bloomington, IN 47403
www.iuniverse.com
1-800-Authors (1-800-288-4677)

Because of the dynamic nature of the Internet, any web addresses or links contained in this book may have changed since publication and may no longer be valid. The views expressed in this work are solely those of the author and do not necessarily reflect the views of the publisher, and the publisher hereby disclaims any responsibility for them.

Any people depicted in stock imagery provided by Getty Images are models, and such images are being used for illustrative purposes only. Certain stock imagery © Getty Images.

ISBN: 978-1-5320-4156-3 (sc)
ISBN: 978-1-5320-4157-0 (e)

Library of Congress Control Number: 2018900709

Printed in the United States of America.

iUniverse rev. date: 08/10/2018

Contents

About the Authors

Joshua C. Klapow is a licensed Clinical Psychologist, behavioral scientist, and human performance coach. He is an Associate Professor of Public Health at The University of Alabama at Birmingham. Dr. Klapow is the author of more than 100 professional articles, abstracts, and book chapters in the area of behavioral medicine and health psychology. He works extensively with local and national media outlets as a Psychological Correspondent to provide expert commentary on the role of psychological, behavioral, and social factors across a broad range of news topics. Dr. Klapow brings psychological insights to topics including health and well-being, mental health, sports, politics, crisis and disaster, parenting, relationships and more. He is the co-host of "The Web with Kurre and Klapow," on Cumulus radio 99.5FM WZRR. "The Web" is an energetic, interactive nightly radio show that explores the challenges and frustrations of love relationships. Dr. Klapow is the Lifestyle Performance Coach for the award-winning Mountain Trek Fitness Retreat and Health Spa.

Dr. Klapow received his Ph.D. in clinical psychology with a specialization in Behavioral Medicine from the University of California, San Diego in 1995. He also completed a fellowship in Geropsychiatry at the University of California, San Diego in 1996.

Sheri D. Pruitt is a licensed Clinical Psychologist with over 25 years of experience. For 16 years, she was Director of Behavioral Science Integration at Kaiser Permanente. Dr. Pruitt guided all behavioral change efforts in the Sacramento Area medical centers, creating large scale programs for physicians, employees, and patients alike. She was a pioneer in digital health and the use of technology for behavioral change. Earlier in her career, Dr. Pruitt worked as a scientist for the World Health Organization where she developed award-winning global models of care for chronic conditions and was principal author of two books. She also spent several years on the faculty of the University of California, San Diego, School of Medicine during which she gained extensive experience in research, publishing, and graduate level education. She has maintained a private consulting practice throughout much of her career and is now focused exclusively on helping organizations meet their health and financial goals through the behavioral change of employees, customers, patients, and administrators.

Dr. Pruitt holds a Bachelor of Science and Master of Education (Summa Cum Laude) from the University of Oklahoma, a Master of Science (with distinction) and a Doctorate from the University of New Mexico with a specialization in Clinical and Health psychology. She is a popular lecturer, trainer, and keynote speaker on the topics of health and wellness, motivation, and the necessity of evidence-based interventions. She frequently shares behavioral science expertise with local and national media outlets.

Acknowledgments

Many people have supported our efforts in writing this book; our patients, students, mentors, and colleagues have all helped to shape its contents. We are also grateful to Arlene Mickley, who helped us navigate the world of publishing.

Our mentors, Mark Slater, Ph.D., Douglas Ferraro, Ph.D., and William R. Miller, Ph.D. helped us develop as scientists and as individuals. We rely daily on the foundation of knowledge they provided.

We also acknowledge and honor the work of Jeffrey Fisher, Ph.D. and William Fisher, Ph.D., whose Information-Motivation-Behavioral Skills model gave us the inspiration and empirical foundation to explain behavior change in a simpler, more intuitive way.

Special thanks to our families, who tolerated endless discussions about titles and graphics, and read numerous drafts. Josh especially thanks his wife, Julie, and his children, Maxwell and Adair. As always, Sheri thanks her parents and her husband, Steve.

To all of us who have ever struggled with the process of change.

Preface

We want to start by setting the record straight. Somehow, despite the many advances in medicine during the past few decades, we have taken a dangerous path when it comes to our health. Obesity is common, lifestyle-related diseases, such as diabetes, are on the increase, and many of us avoid healthy behaviors, such as following a healthy diet, exercising, taking medication properly, getting adequate sleep, not smoking, and reducing the stress in our lives. We are searching and hoping for a pill, surgery, or procedure that will make us healthy—quickly and with little effort.

When it comes to such things as a headache, an upset stomach, or a bacterial infection, often there is a quick fix. But we absolutely must stop this line of thinking when it comes to health-related lifestyles. Every step we take to improve our health requires that we change our behavior. There is no magic bullet or a way to make changes that requires nothing from us. The reality is that change requires each person to put forth some amount of effort.

A great deal is known about how to make needed changes in health-related behavior—or any other behavior, for that matter. Theories of behavioral change such as the "Transtheoretical Model of Behavior Change," the "Health Belief Model," the "Theory of Planned Behavior," and "Social Learning Theory" have all proposed reasonable explanations as to how and why behavior change occurs.

The problem with these theories and the impression they give to the general public is that changing behavior is either

- ➢ Incredibly complicated, and dependent on a series of cognitive, emotional, and behavioral interactions that may require professional counseling; or
- ➢ A simple matter of common sense and self-motivation.

We believe there is a lot of room between these two extremes. This book will give you a set of tools that goes beyond "common sense and motivation," without attempting to deal with the complexities of psychological treatment and advanced behavioral science. Why? Because most of the answers to making healthy lifestyle changes can be found somewhere in between. We like the common sense, the simplicity, and the scientific foundation of the Information-Motivation-Behavioral Skills model of change developed by Jeffrey Fisher, Ph.D. and his brother, William Fisher, Ph.D. We use their model as the basis for a simple set of guiding principles that will give you the ability to change any health behavior or health habit.

What a powerful concept. This book will help you take control of your health and your life. The information it contains works with any diet, exercise, sleep, or stop-smoking program. In fact, this book will help you change any behavior that has a negative impact on your well-being, health-related or not.

The essential tools you need to make change happen are the SMART skills, a set of self-management skills, which underlie all successful behavior change. SMART is an acronym that can help you remember these skills:

Set a goal
Monitor your progress
Arrange your world for success
Recruit a support team
Treat yourself

Living SMART is based on the idea that your health and well-being is determined mostly by what you do or don't do every day. Regardless of the severity of your situation, the history of the problems or how complicated the issue may feel, your success is determined by the actions you take. This set of principles will guide you through the process of change. Living SMART means:

➢ Having the skills to change what you need to change and what you want to change.
➢ Not being perfect, but doing the "right" behaviors more days than not.
➢ Having the confidence that you can succeed.

If you keep the acronym SMART in mind and use the skills it represents, you will be well on your way to making lasting changes in your lifestyle.

In our work, we talk to patients, health care professionals, executive boards, human resource professionals, local reading clubs, college students, and many others. Two things have become clear to us from these experiences. First, people are pleasantly surprised to find that changing their behavior doesn't have to be an arduous task. Second, they are usually quite busy and welcome help and guidance with the change process. We took these two facts to heart in writing this book.

Living SMART can be read in sections. You don't need to read it from cover to cover to get what you need. Read Part I: "What It Takes to Change Your Health" if you want to understand the basic principles that underlie making any change in behavior. Sometimes we need a little extra guidance to "jump start" our progress towards change.

Having a game plan or strategy is critical. Diet, exercise, taking medications, and getting adequate sleep are common health-related behaviors that have a huge impact on overall health and well-being. Because these are such common issues, we'll give you a strategy for making changes in each of them. The information in Part II: "Your Game Plans" will help you start making changes in any or all of these areas.

"When Life Gets Tough" in Part III (Chapter 11) can help you when you are having problems sticking with the changes you've made, as everyone does. If you need a quick tip, something to help you with a current concern, take a look at the "Action Tips" found throughout each chapter with more listed in Chapter 12. The Appendix includes some reminders, forms and charts, and more details about changing eating and exercising behaviors.

We are excited about this book, and enthusiastic about helping you become as healthy as possible. But remember, it's what you do or don't do every day that affects your health more than anything else. Take control now and become healthier starting today. Here's to your health!

Joshua C. Klapow, Ph.D.
Sheri D. Pruitt, Ph.D.

Introduction
Stop Wishing and Start Living SMART

Congratulations on wanting to be healthy. You are taking an important step by reading this book, which will tell you exactly how to change your behavior to improve your health and change your lifestyle.

The Problem: Our Health

You've probably noticed we're in big trouble in our country. Obesity is at an all-time high, diabetes is skyrocketing, and only half of us take our medications the way our doctors prescribe. People are still smoking, drinking too much, and sleeping too little. We're more stressed out and more sedentary than ever before. How can this be? We have the most sophisticated healthcare system in the world—the best doctors, the most medications. Why are Americans so unhealthy?

The Reason: Our Behavior

We are the reason that we're unhealthy. Every one of us has some level of control over our own health, but we've been ignoring the root of so many of our health problems: our behavior.

With all the talk about increasing health care costs, chronic disease, and diseases caused by lifestyle, there has been little discussion about how people can change their habits to improve their health. We've heard that health habits are important and that we should change them, but how?

The degree to which our behavior affects our health often surprises people. In our work as psychologists, people often ask us about genetics. They say: "Don't genes determine a person's health?" Genetics are important. Your genes set the stage for how behavior affects your health. Think of your genes as the hand of cards you have been dealt. If you have a good set of genes, you can do unhealthy things and still live well. If you were born with a set of genes that make you susceptible to health issues, you need to make the effort to be as healthy as possible, because the cards are stacked against you.

Consider heart disease. It has a genetic component, but behavior can dramatically influence its development. If you have genes that make you susceptible to heart disease and you smoke, drink too much, and never exercise, what will happen? You'll most likely develop serious heart problems. If you have the same genes and you keep your weight in check, exercise, drink in moderation, and don't smoke, you may never have heart problems. We can say the same thing about diabetes, obesity, and many other conditions.

Changing Behavior: It's Not Just about Being Motivated

You've been told to get motivated and make changes in your lifestyle, right? Not so fast! As psychologists, we see patients every day who are frustrated and sick, and getting sicker. They've been told to change their diet, relax, exercise, and stop smoking and drinking. When they fail to make these necessary changes, they're told they lack motivation. People look everywhere for answers about how to change: the Internet, self-help books, magazines, and infomercials, but they can't find the solution.

There are scientific answers to this problem. Psychologists and others who study human behavior have known for decades what it takes to successfully change health habits. However, the answers they've come up with haven't been readily available to the people who need them—or when the answers are available, they have been presented in ways that are difficult to understand and apply to daily life.

We All Need a Healthier Lifestyle

Whether you want to start an exercise program, begin to diet, quit smoking, reduce stress, get more organized, spend less money, or make any other lifestyle change, many books and programs are available. The sheer number of different strategies can be overwhelming, but there is a common thread: All of the diet and exercise books, the stop-smoking programs, and the organizational and financial strategies require that you change your behavior in order to succeed.

Unfortunately, these tools often lack instructions on how to change your behavior. Most of the information about improving lifestyle focuses only on what to change, rarely on how to change. This is the missing piece that makes the difference between success and failure when it comes to changing health-related behavior. The information in Living SMART works with any diet, exercise, or stop-smoking program. It gives you what the others do not: a simple approach to change any behavior that has a negative impact on your health and lifestyle

Myth and Reality

Many false claims, myths, and erroneous assumptions have helped to create a way of thinking that is counterproductive. For example:

➢ Myth: If I just want to badly enough, I can make improvements in my health.
➢ Truth: This is the reason people fail. Motivation can only take you so far; it goes up and it goes down. You can't rely on it alone. Without the skills to make the changes you desire, you will not succeed in the long run.
➢ Myth: This behavior change stuff doesn't apply to me. My problem is more complicated.
➢ Truth: Anyone who wants to be healthier needs to change their habits. Regardless of the severity of your problems or your level of physical impairment, improving your health requires doing some things and not doing others. Whether it's taking medication, following your doctor's recommendations, or monitoring blood pressure, you will have to do something differently than you have done before.
➢ Myth: Changing behavior is just common sense.
➢ Truth: Our approach is so straightforward and so simple that people think it's not powerful. In reality, you can change any behavior if you have the right information and some motivation, and use the SMART skills. If you are struggling, you are probably missing one or more of the basic principles of change outlined in this book.
➢ Myth: I tried this before and it didn't work.
➢ Truth: You either didn't use the principles and skills, or—as is more often the case—you used them for a period of time, hit a roadblock, and then stopped. Living healthier does not mean being perfect. It means adopting healthy habits more days than not. If everyone were to have this perspective, we would all enjoy better health.
➢ Myth: I really want to be healthy; I just don't have the motivation.
➢ Truth: If you want to be healthy, then you already have some level of motivation. You may not have enough to carry you through to reach your goal right now, but you are definitely motivated enough to get started.

- ➤ Myth: If I just understood what caused my bad habits, I could change them.
- ➤ Truth: Understanding how your habits developed, and why they developed, is important because it can keep you from repeating a destructive pattern. However, understanding why your bad habits developed is not enough to help you change them. Living healthier means adopting a simple set of principles and skills, and using them to guide your behavior more often than not. No one is perfect.

Okay—the myths are behind us. Are you ready to live a healthier life? Let's go!

The Icons for Important Themes

Our goal in writing this book was to make it as simple, straightforward, and useful as possible. Thus, we have included icons as well as words to communicate efficiently and signal important themes. The icons found throughout the book are illustrated below.

This icon signals research findings, scientific principles, or technical terms.

This icon signals an interactive exercise that requires your response.

This icon signals key points and our recommendations.

PART 1

What It Takes to Change Your Health

You have to start somewhere—you need a base from which you can begin to work. This section lays out the principles you need in order to understand what goes into making changes in your lifestyle. The ideas presented here are drawn from the work of Jeffrey Fisher, Ph.D. and William Fisher, Ph.D., whose Information-Motivation-Behavioral Skills model (Fisher & Fisher, 1992) gave us the inspiration and empirical foundation to explain behavior change in a simpler, more intuitive way.

This section will be your foundation for any change you wish to make. It outlines the necessary elements for change and is a framework for understanding how change comes about.

1

Let's Get Started

At one time or another, most of us have tried to improve our health by changing our behavior, often without success. Maybe you've tried to stop smoking, lose weight, or exercise regularly. If you haven't been successful yet, don't be too hard on yourself. True behavior change requires three important components. We call them "The What," "The Want," and "The How." Chances are you're simply missing one of them. When it comes to changing behavior, most people fall into one of three groups, or "change types."

What Is Your "Change Type?"

1.   Uninformed: "I don't know what to do to be healthy." Do you know what you need to do to feel your best? For example, are you aware that exercising, eating right, and following your doctor's recommendations are good for your health? Do you know the amount and type of exercise to do? Do you know the number of calories you should be eating? Do you know what your doctor has advised you to do to take care of yourself? Most people answer "yes" to these questions. If your answer is "yes," move on to the next category.

   If your answer is "no," you might be "uninformed," or need more accurate information about the behaviors you need to change, but you can easily get the details about what you need to do to be healthy.

2.   Unmotivated: "I don't want to do anything differently in order to improve my health." Do you want to behave in a way that will ensure that you are healthy and feel your best? Most people answer "yes" to this question—it's the "I know exercise is good for me and I want to do it" category. Move on to the third category if you answered "yes."

If you answered "no," you probably already know all about exercise, and understand that being active has great health benefits, but you just don't feel like exercising. You don't really want to do anything differently to get more activity into your daily routine, although you know it would make you feel better. Many people find themselves in this place at one time or another. Motivation fluctuates. It changes depending on the behavior, the setting, and even the day! If you don't feel very motivated, don't worry. We will give you some ways to tap into your internal motivation to be healthier.

3. Unskilled: "I don't know how to make changes in my behavior." You know what health behaviors are good for you, and you want to make those behaviors part of your life, but you just can't seem to do it. People in this category lack the skills they need to make effective lifestyle changes. Do you know how to make healthy behaviors part of your everyday life? If your answer is "no" or "I'm not sure," you are similar to most of us. Few people know how to incorporate healthy behaviors into their lifestyles, even though they understand that making changes will help them feel better and they want to make them.

The typical response of health professionals is to tell clients over and over again that exercise (or another healthy behavior) is good for them, or that they simply need to be more motivated. However, neither of these responses seems to help people change.

These three categories don't only apply to exercise. They work for virtually any health-related behavior. People usually fall into one of the three categories no matter what behavior they want to change, including dieting, smoking, taking medication, wearing a seat belt, or checking their blood pressure on a regular basis. In this chapter, you will learn the basic principles for making healthy lifestyle changes.

The Principles of Change

The ability to change your behavior in order to create a healthier lifestyle comes down to three critical factors: knowing what to do, wanting to do it, and knowing how to do it. It's really as simple as it sounds. You need The What, The Want, and The How to make any behavior change.

The What:

The What is information. You need to know what changes to make in order to reach your health goal; for example, what exercise, what food, or what medications to take at what doses.

The Want:

The Want is motivation. You need to find some amount of internal motivation to change, plain and simple.

The How:

The How includes the skills you need to be able to change. You need to know how to make changes in your behavior so you can reach your goal. Many of us are missing these essential skills.

Research has shown that changing health behavior requires more than motivation—information and skills are also necessary (Fisher & Fisher, 2000; Fisher et al, 2003; Chang et al, 2014).

In our society, we make two big assumptions about changing health behaviors. We believe that people who succeed do so because they want to, and that those who fail just aren't motivated. Or we think that if we know what behaviors we need to practice (such as dieting, exercising, reducing stress, or stopping smoking), and are motivated to do them, we will be successful at making changes.

If these assumptions are true, you have to wonder whether we have a country filled with uninformed, unmotivated people. Maybe so, but we believe there is another explanation. Think about your exercise habits for a minute and then answer these questions.

1. Have you heard that exercising three to five times a week, for at least 30 minutes, is good for your health?

   YES   NO

2. Do you want exercise to be a part of your lifestyle?

   YES   NO

3. Do you exercise three to five times per week for 30 minutes or more, and have you done so consistently for the past 6 months?

   YES   NO

Where are you lacking? Is it that you don't know? You're not motivated? Or, you don't have a skill set to ensure you can exercise consistently? Most people are missing skills and skills are something that everyone can learn.

Three Simple Steps to Change

Any time you want to make a health change, all you need to do is determine which of the three ingredients (The What, The Want, or The How) is missing. Ask yourself these questions:

1. The What:

    Do you know exactly what behavior to change? For example, what exercise do I need to do for how long, what food or how many calories should I eat, or what medications should I take and at what doses?

2. The Want:

    How important is it that you make the change? How motivated are you to do it?

3. The How:

    Do you know how to change your behavior to reach your lifestyle goal?

Where Do I Start?

Next, use your answers to these questions to jump-start your behavioral change. If you answered "no" to question # 1, you need to gather information. Chapter 2 will be useful in helping you find what you need. If you answered "no" to question # 2, then you need to find your motivation. Chapter 3 will give you some tips on enhancing your desire to do things differently. Finally, if you answered "no" to question # 3, you need to learn how to change your behavior. Chapter 4 has the answers. It really is that simple.

SMART Skills—The Key to "The How"

The core principle of this book is that you need to develop what we call "SMART" skills to make the change happen. SMART is an acronym for these five essential skills:

Set a goal
Monitor your progress
Arrange your world for success
Recruit a support team
Treat yourself

Throughout this book, we'll explain each skill in detail. Are you ready to get started?

ACTION TIP

Exercise for People Who Hate Exercise

We all know that daily exercise is good for our health. But what if you just hate it? What if you can't stand the thought of jogging, lifting weights, or doing aerobics? Try these suggestions:

➢ Identify one small physical activity that you can do without much effort. Maybe you could walk up and down the stairs every day, or walk for 5 minutes around the neighborhood. The easier the activity, the better to help you get started.
➢ Write down what you plan to do and post it on the fridge.
➢ Commit to doing this activity for one week. At the end of the week, decide if you want to continue and, hopefully, do more.

Once you engage in a small amount of activity on a regular basis, you can gradually increase your efforts as you feel successful and your confidence grows. With time it will become easier and part of your routine.

2

The What: Know Exactly What Needs to Change

Information is essential when making any lifestyle change. You need it to get started. If you don't know what you need to change, all the motivation and behavioral skills in the world won't help you. Information is without a doubt the easiest of the three ingredients to obtain. When it comes to exercise, diet, stress management, diabetes care, obesity, smoking—you name it—a wealth of information is available.

If you're reading this, you probably already know what behavioral change you need to make. However, people tend to focus all of their efforts on getting more and more information. They assume that the more information they have about making changes, the more likely they are to make them. This is simply not so. You need accurate information about the behavior you want to change. You don't need to be an expert on the topic.

Time and again, research has shown that information alone is not enough to change health behaviors. Smokers know that smoking is bad for their health, but they continue to smoke anyway. People who are overweight know they should shed the extra pounds, but they remain heavy. We are bombarded with information about health—we all know what to do. If information was the answer, we would all be totally healthy. Information is necessary, but not powerful enough on its own to help you change (Mazucca, 1982).

Any information you gather must be reliable and useful. The quality and accuracy of the information is important, not the quantity. A quick and easy way to organize your sources is to break them down into categories, as we've done here.

Sources of Information

People. Ask your doctor about any behaviors related to your health. Whether the topic is exercise, diet, blood-sugar monitoring, preventive tests, or psychological problems and counseling, your doctor's job is to support you in your quest to be healthier. Realize, however, that in today's healthcare setting your doctor may not have the time to provide you with a comprehensive education on all health topics. Rather, she may refer you to another healthcare professional or to another source of information. Either way, consulting with your doctor about lifestyle changes is a good way to begin.

Prepare yourself before you go to the doctor. Remember, you may only have a few minutes to discuss lifestyle changes. Prepare for the visit by doing the following:

➢ Write your questions on a piece of paper and take it with you to the office visit.
➢ Organize the questions in order of importance. You may not have time to ask them all, so this will ensure that the most important ones are answered.
➢ When you call for an appointment, tell the doctor or office staff that you have some specific questions about lifestyle changes.
➢ Bring a pen and paper to take notes.

Written Information. The number of books, magazines, reports, and Internet sources on health is overwhelming. No one source is the most accurate, up-to-date, or reliable. When it comes to analyzing written resources, follow these general rules:

➢ Credibility. The information should come from a respected institution or organization. Here are just a few examples:
  - Universities, such as Johns Hopkins, Harvard, or UCLA
  - Government agencies, such as the National Institutes of Health/National Library of Medicine, Centers for Disease Control, and the Department of Health and Human Services
  - Disease-specific organizations, such as the American Heart Association or American Cancer Society
  - Healthcare systems, such as The Mayo Clinic or Kaiser Permanente

➤ Timeliness. Look at the date of publication to make sure that the information is current. In general, it's best to collect information that is no more than 5 years old.

➤ Consistency. Check to see that the information is consistent across a variety of sources. Conflicting views may pop up, but the information should be similar.

➤ Trustworthiness. If it sounds too good to be true, it probably is. Use common sense when evaluating information. Just because a publication uses terms you don't understand, it doesn't mean you can't grasp the overall message. Words such as "miracle," "instant," and "guaranteed" should be warning flags.

Mass Media. The same rules apply to television and radio. The source should be credible, the information should be consistent, and the claims should be reasonable. It's important to note that television and radio sources of health information can be incredibly brief. A 30-second public service announcement, a 3-minute news report, or a 10-minute radio segment may not give the whole story. While the information may be accurate, it probably won't give you the whole picture. Think of radio and television as good starting points from which to gather facts or ideas for further pursuit.

There are many other available resources that can help you better understand the behavior you want or need to change. Google your topic. Information is at your fingertips. Getting what you need should be simple. Remember, you need information about the lifestyle *behavior* you want to change. Now, let's move on to the more challenging components of change: The Want and The How.

3

The Want: Decide Whether You Want to Change

Motivation—or lack thereof—is the great stumbling block. "If only I were motivated enough, I could do this." Negative thoughts, self-defeating beliefs, and a history of failed attempts at making changes all contribute to decreased self-esteem, diminished self-efficacy, and low motivation. Why do you have negative thoughts and beliefs? What is driving them? Although the answers to these questions are important, not having answers doesn't mean you can't change your unwanted behaviors. Many books focus on the origin of self-defeating thoughts, attitudes, and beliefs; countless magazine articles focus on why you think the way you do. These sources can help, but they may not be completely necessary. We often spend so much time focusing on why we are the way we are that we don't focus on moving forward. Motivation is complicated, but we can simplify it by getting right to the heart of the question. Ask yourself, "How important is it that I make a change in my behavior?" In other words, how important is it to do something differently to improve your health?

If your answer to this question is: "Changing my behavior to improve my health is not important to me," you're not going to make the change successfully. Sometimes people are not ready emotionally or psychologically to do things differently. If you are absolutely not ready to change, nothing can force you to do it. However, if you are even slightly motivated to do something differently, you can have success. With just a small amount of motivation, you can take action and that action may boost your level of motivation and confidence enough to keep you moving forward.

Evaluate your level of motivation using this scale:

| 1 | 2 | 3 | 4 | 5 | 6 | 7 | 8 | 9 | 10 |

Not motivated   Strongly motivated

Your motivation level may be higher or lower depending on the activity, the time, and the setting. The most important thing is to have some motivation to get beyond not doing anything. Once you find it, you can boost your motivation when necessary. This chapter includes several strategies to help you do just that. So, stop worrying about motivation—chances are you'll find enough inside to succeed. Below are some ideas to help you.

Think about Your Future

What if you aren't sure you are motivated enough to make a change? What if you think it's not worth it to be healthier? Stop for a minute and think about your future. If you don't change your lifestyle, will you still be here 5 years from now? Will you be in any kind of shape to work, go on vacation, and enjoy life? How will you feel? What will you look like? Your future and your ability to do the things you enjoy in that future are determined mostly by what you do today, tomorrow, the next day, and so on.

Consider the Relationship between Your Behavior and Your Health

Do you want to make the lifestyle changes that are necessary to be healthy? If you're not sure, ask yourself these questions and write down the answers

> ➤ What concerns do you have about your health?

_____.

> ➤ What things are you currently doing to be healthier?

_____.

> ➤ If you could make some improvements in your health, how would you feel?

_____.

> ➤ What else would be different about you?

_____.

➢ What would be better for your loved ones if you made health improvements?

_____.

➢ What behavior have you been able to successfully change in the past?

_____.

➢ When do you plan to get started?

_____.

By taking the time to answer these questions, you will be able to tap into your personal reasons for wanting to change (Miller and Rollnick 2013). Later on, these answers will be reminders of why you set out to make changes in the first place. Simple as it seems, these little prompts can really boost your level of motivation along the way. So, if you ever find your motivation slipping, review your answers or repeat this exercise.

How Important Is Change? Can I Do It?

Using the scales below, rate how important it is for you to make the behavioral change you're considering and how confident you are that you will succeed.

1. How important is it that I make the change?

    1   2   3   4   5   6   7   8   9   10

    Not important   Extremely important

2. What would make this behavioral change more important?

    _____

    _____

3. Am I confident I can make the change?

   1   2   3   4   5   6   7   8   9   10

   Not confident   Extremely confident

4. What would make you more confident?

   _____

   _____

After answering all of these questions, you have probably discovered a number of reasons for wanting to change an unhealthy behavior. You may have noticed that your emotions play a significant role in your decision to make the change. Thinking about changing a behavior can bring up a variety of feelings, including anger, fear of failure, and anxiety. While change can be difficult and stressful, consider the consequences of refusing to change. What are you doing today to become the healthy person you envision yourself being in the future? How long can you afford to wait before making the change?

A Possible Shortcut around Motivation

Do you have thoughts similar to these?

➢ "I just don't have any willpower."
➢ "If I only knew why I undermine myself."
➢ "All of my problems stem from my mother" (a psychologist joke!).

This kind of "self-talk" is a psychological merry-go-round that can keep you from changing your behavior. However, there may be a way to get off this carnival ride. It's possible to change your thoughts, emotions, and your level of motivation by first changing your behavior, because changing behavior has a way of changing the way we see ourselves.

It's difficult to think of yourself as failing at exercise when you are walking for 30 minutes, four times a week. It's hard to say you're not confident in your ability to diet when you have cut down on the amount of sweets you eat. Get the new behavior going and your confidence and perceptions will follow!

ACTION TIP

Unclutter Your Life

Ugh—clutter—it's everywhere and it seems to grow and grow. Most of us want to get organized, but it can be stressful and overwhelming. Where do you start? How long will it take? The key to getting clutter out of your life is to start small, very small.

For clutter at home, don't try to organize your whole house or even a whole room. Instead, chose one small section of a room to organize. Then, pick a day and a set amount of time to get the job done. When you've got the first section done, chose another. Same thing at work; tackle office clutter one corner at a time. Remember, it took weeks or maybe even years to accumulate that clutter. Tackling the job, one section at time, will make the task much more manageable and a lot less stressful. When you participate in the behaviors you want to adopt, it is difficult to see yourself as a failure.

Dealing with Negative Thoughts

You can be sailing along and, all of a sudden, it happens. Some small setback occurs in your diet, exercise program, or management of your blood pressure, and then the flood of negative thoughts comes. Negative thoughts and feelings will dampen your motivation, but they don't have to mean the end of your success. You can manage them before they take over. Here is a simple three-step strategy to manage negative thoughts:

1. Notice when you have negative thoughts. Negative thoughts usually follow a slip-up in maintaining a changed behavior—you strayed from your diet or you missed your workout. Take a minute to write down what's going through your mind. What are your thoughts? What are you saying to yourself? Maybe you're thinking: "I have no self-control" or "I'm not disciplined enough to do this."

2. Turn the thought into an action. Once you've caught the negative thought and written it down, repeat it out loud, but imagine that someone else is saying it to you. For example, imagine that someone said, "You have no self-control" or "You're just not disciplined enough." As silly as this may sound, you will be more likely to stick up for yourself by picturing someone else saying the words to you.

3. Defend yourself. Is it really true that you have no self-control? Chances are this negative thought isn't 100% accurate. Write down as many situations as you can think of that prove this negative thought is wrong. Think about the times when you have shown self-control. Also, think about other explanations for why you slipped up this time. The bottom line is to defend yourself against the negative thought.

This exercise won't keep you from having negative thoughts, and it won't prevent occasional slip-ups, but it can help keep negative thoughts from taking over and ruining your efforts. By being aware of negative thoughts as they come up, and working to manage them, you will be more likely to stay motivated and stay on track with the behaviors that are important to you.

Still Not Motivated?

After going through these exercises, most people are reminded of why they want to make changes. They find the motivation to do something differently. If you've read this section and gone through the exercises, and you still have no motivation—then we are concerned. Changing does require effort, so it's possible you truly lack the motivation right now to be healthier. Perhaps you feel you'll be okay without making changes. Perhaps you simply don't want to change your lifestyle or your health. You make the choice. The timing may not be right.

However, most people are ready to take the next step: learning the SMART skills you will need to make changes in your health behavior. The next chapter will help you do just that.

ACTION TIP

Optimism

Did you know that being optimistic can improve your health? Research has shown that optimistic people tend to have stronger immune systems, are less prone to cancer, and tend to live longer following a heart attack. The good news is that optimism is a behavior that can be learned. Try this exercise:

Every night at bedtime, write down three things that went really well during the day. They can be small things such as: "My kids were cooperative and gave me a hug," or big things: "Today I got a raise" or "I got promoted." Next to each event, write down the reasons why the good thing happened. For example, maybe your children were cooperative because they went to bed earlier the night before. Doing this exercise will help you spend part of your day thinking about and focusing on positive events in your life, and you will end your day on an optimistic note. Over time, you will begin to increase your level of optimism. Why not start being more optimistic—it's good for you, and it will benefit the people around you, too.

4

The How: SMART Skills to Change Your Behavior

Remember the five SMART skills:

Set a goal
Monitor your progress
Arrange your world for success
Recruit a support team
Treat yourself

Here comes the part that gets over-looked, swept under the carpet, or written off as "just common sense." The secret is that for most people, these SMART skills are the key to being successful. When they fail to use the skills, they struggle; when they use them, they succeed. There's nothing magic about this—these are skills that everyone can learn and they are based on the results from decades of behavioral science research. One problem is that people don't use the skills because they seem so simple and straightforward. They are often discounted because people think there must be more to it. Please hear us loud and clear on this one—surrender to the simplicity of SMART skills! If you know what needs to change and you are motivated to make the change, with these five skills you will succeed.

Why the acronym SMART? This acronym is simply to help you remember to be SMART about changing your behavior. Use SMART to remember the set of skills that are needed to make any change. If you learn and adopt these skills, you will be able to change any behavior. As we have seen, even those who are highly motivated to change often fail because changing is more than simply wanting to change; it also requires information and a set of essential skills.

Behavioral skills are nothing more than self-management techniques that increase your chances of changing your behavior. Think about learning them in the same way as you might think about learning how to play a sport or musical instrument. For example, to play basketball you need to be able to run, jump, dribble, shoot, and pass. You may know quite a bit about the sport of basketball, but without these basic skills you won't be successful in playing it. In addition, you can't be successful at basketball if you only know how to dribble or pass. To play the sport you need all of the skills.

Apply this concept to making lifestyle changes. If you want to eat differently, exercise, stop smoking, reduce stress, or make any other change, you need a set of skills to be successful. This is where the SMART skills come in. These techniques should be used together to achieve change. They will help you make any change you want, but only if you apply all of them. It's that simple. The first SMART skill is:

Set a Goal

Think for a moment about a trip or vacation you took recently. Did you decide where you wanted to go before you left? Did you decide how you were going to get there? Of course you did! Making plans is simple common sense. Basic plans such as these are also the foundation of goal-setting. Goal-setting involves establishing where you want to go and how you plan to get there. As the saying goes, "Most people don't plan to fail, they fail to plan."

How do you set the right goal? Goals such as "I want to exercise daily," "I want to lose weight," or "I want to get more sleep," are good ideas, but they are not specific enough. When you think about setting goals, keep two words in mind: "observable" and "measurable." Take a second and think about this. It's difficult to observe "exercise," but you can easily observe specific types of exercise such as walking, running, swimming, or weight lifting. You can't observe diet, but you can observe the specific foods and calories you consume. You can't observe getting more sleep, but you can observe the number of hours of sleep you get each night. By making your goals observable, they automatically become measurable. The basic idea is that if you can see it, you can measure it. Once your goals are measurable you can chart them, keep track of them, and bingo! You have a road map from your starting point to your end point.

ACTION TIP

Stay on Top of Your Healthy Assets

What do balancing your checkbook and staying healthy have in common? We all know that balancing our checkbook helps us keep track of money so we don't overspend. The same principle applies to virtually any health habit. By tracking your health habits, you'll automatically increase your chances for a healthier life.

Writing down what you do will increase your chances of sticking with a diet or exercise program, or remembering to take your medication. Every time you exercise, write down what you did, the day you did it, and the amount of time you exercised. If you are dieting, simply jot down everything you eat in a notebook you keep with you. If you are taking medications, keep a calendar to track the times you take it. The same applies to any lifestyle behavior you are trying to change.

We call the observable and measurable behaviors you want to accomplish "target behaviors."

One of the biggest problems people have in trying to change their behavior is that they don't specify their target behaviors. Think about brushing your teeth. Seems simple enough, right? Now think about teaching a 3-year-old child how to brush his teeth. Remember, this is as foreign to him as learning a new language might be to you. How would you do it? You could just "show" him by modeling it. But that usually doesn't work. A better approach would be to break down the simple task of brushing his teeth into even smaller steps; for example:

1. Unscrew the top of the toothpaste.
2. Pick up the toothbrush.
3. Hold the toothbrush in one hand and squeeze the toothpaste onto the toothbrush with the other hand.
4. Put the toothpaste down.
5. Turn on the water.

6. Put the toothbrush under the water for 3 seconds.
7. Raise the toothbrush to your mouth.
8. Brush each tooth in a slow, circular motion.
9. Spit out the excess toothpaste into the sink.
10. Rinse off the toothbrush.
11. Fill a small cup with water.
12. Take a small amount of water into your mouth and swish it around.
13. Spit out the water.
14. Turn the water off.
15. Wipe your mouth.
16. Replace the top of the toothpaste tube cap.
17. Put the toothpaste and toothbrush away.

The simpler the behavior, the greater the chance you have of accomplishing it. Brushing teeth maybe confusing for a 3-year-old, but each one of these 17 tasks alone is quite manageable. Break the act down into simple tasks, and the child will succeed.

Let's now bring this concept back to lifestyle changes. Adults, too, need help with breaking big tasks into manageable pieces. Below are some examples of general goals and corresponding target behaviors that are observable and measurable:

General Goal	Target Behavior
1. I want to eat better.	I will eat five servings of fruits or vegetables each day.
2. I want to exercise more.	I will walk every day, starting at 15 minutes a day and increasing by 5 minutes a week until I am walking 30 minutes each day.
3. I need to relax.	I will practice relaxation exercises for 5 minutes, three times a day (before breakfast, after lunch, and before bedtime).

To make any lifestyle change, you must start with a goal. Chances are that goal will be too broad at first. So, break your goal down into its smallest target behaviors.

Let's practice the first step toward reaching your goals. Below, write down three of your general health goals and then break each one down into target behaviors that you can see and measure.

General Health Goal   Target Behaviors

1. _____   _____

   _____   _____

   _____   _____

2. _____   _____

   _____   _____

   _____   _____

3. _____   _____

   _____   _____

   _____   _____

Your goal should be observable, measurable, and something you feel confident that you can achieve.

So how do you decide the level at which to set your goal? Most people have a tendency to shoot for the stars, even when they break their goals down into target behaviors. If you want to be able to exercise 5 days a week, you already know that you must break the exercise down into specific target behaviors. Let's say your target behavior is to lift weights for 20 minutes and walk for 20 minutes, 5 days a week, but you haven't been very active over the last few years. Should you start out at this level? Think about what might happen if you do.

You make it through the full workout on the first day. You're pretty tired and wake up the next day feeling sore, fatigued, and generally worn out. What are you likely to do? You probably feel too tired to go back and do it again. You decide to skip a day, because you still have 5 days left in the week to get in four more workouts. You work out again the next day, but you're still sore and unable to complete the 20-minute walking portion of the workout. The next morning, you wake up fatigued and still sore.

Where are you at this point? You've successfully completed one workout, skipped another, and partially completed a second. You are not on a good path. Your workouts are already becoming spotty, and each one is followed by unpleasant consequences (feeling sore and fatigued). You probably don't feel good about yourself or your ability to be successful.

Behaviors that do not produce consistently positive results are not likely to be repeated. To make your new behavior a habit, you need to guarantee that each workout has a good chance of being a success. This is where pacing comes in. Pacing is simply the act of gradually increasing the intensity, duration, and frequency of a desired behavior in a way that maximizes your chances of success.

Whether your goal is a 40-minute walk or the elimination of excess salt from your diet, pacing can help you accomplish it. The rule of thumb is that making gradual changes toward your goal are more likely to lead to success than one giant change. For any given health behavior, ask yourself this question: "What portion of the behavior am I absolutely sure I can do successfully?" or "What target behavior am I sure I can achieve?"

ACTION TIP

Pace Yourself

Developing any health habit starts with setting a specific goal. But even if your goal is specific, you can get into trouble if it isn't reachable right from the start. An hour of running every day, or trying to lose 30 pounds in 2 weeks, may be more than you can handle. If you can't do the behavior consistently, you'll never reach the goal. The trick is to pace yourself.

Using exercise as an example, let's say you're absolutely sure you can accomplish 30 minutes of walking. Take that amount and cut it in half for the first week. For the first week, you will walk for no more and no less than 15 minutes. For each subsequent week, add 5 more minutes to the workout, no more and no less. At the end of 4 weeks, you will have reached your goal, and you also will have been exercising for 4 weeks. Research shows that, in order to exercise regularly, you must develop the exercise habit before you develop the physical conditioning. You accomplish two things with this pacing schedule: You are practicing the behavior consistently and you are giving yourself the best chance at success each time you practice it. Those two accomplishments are absolutely critical for developing healthy habits.

Remember, it's better to start small and be successful over the long term than to shoot for the stars and miss. You are creating lifelong habits. Set yourself up for success by setting goals you can achieve.

Monitor Your Progress

Sometimes we talk ourselves out of making healthy lifestyle changes. We've all made these types of statements to ourselves: "I didn't eat that much ice cream," "I'll just work out extra hard next time," or "I only had one cigarette yesterday."

Our minds are powerful and great at helping us rationalize unhealthy choices. Changing your lifestyle can be challenging enough, and excuses and rationalizations seem to slip in if the target behaviors are not counted and tracked. Does this mean you aren't motivated? Does it mean that you're a failure? No, it just means that you are trying to break one habit and start another, and your mind is trying to keep things the same as they have always been.

"Self-monitoring" is a technical term for keeping a written record of your journey towards your goal. The detailed monitoring chart—called simply "The Chart"—in Chapter 6 offers a good way to conduct self-monitoring. (The smaller version below is for illustrative purposes only.) The Chart can be used to track any behavior, including eating, exercising, smoking, sleeping, watching television, and taking medication. Not only will self-monitoring help you keep track of what you are doing, it can also have a positive impact on the goal you are trying to achieve. In fact, charting your behavior is what we call a "psychological freebie." It may seem trivial; something that doesn't take much time or effort, but it packs a powerful punch. Monitoring behavior has a way of changing behavior.

The Chart (See Chapter 6 for complete version.)

My desired behavior is:_____.
(Be specific.)
I will practice this behavior_____days per week.
My short-term goal is_____.
My long-term goal is_____.

SUN	MON	TUE	WED	THU	FRI	SAT

Time and again, research has shown that the simple act of monitoring a behavior can change that behavior (Butryn, Phelan, Hill & Wing, 2007). We call this the self-monitoring effect. Behaviors such as exercise, are likely to increase when they are monitored, and behaviors such as eating high-fat foods or smoking, are likely to decrease with monitoring.

Is monitoring the answer to all lifestyle changes? Does it come with a money-back guarantee? Sorry—there are no quick fixes here. Remember, monitoring is just one of the five SMART skills that will help you make changes in your lifestyle. Here's what's behind the "magic."

Monitoring your behavior does several things. First, it puts up a barrier to the tricks your mind can play. It creates a visual account of your actual behavior and puts it in black and white. If you have a blank spot on your chart because you didn't exercise, you will be forced to deal with it. Given this evidence, you will have to consider the reason why you didn't. The same thing goes for the amount of ice cream you ate. Was it a lot? Was it a little? Monitoring eliminates the uncertainty by turning "a lot" or "a little" into an actual measurable amount.

Monitoring is especially important during the early stages of a behavior change because it allows you to stay aware of where you are and recognize problems early on. Monitoring also provides a visual reminder, or cue, for you to practice the behavior. However, your monitoring chart will serve as a visual reminder only if it is kept in a place where you can easily see it. If you place your chart in a desk drawer, it will not have the same effect as placing it in a highly visible location, such as on the refrigerator, the bathroom mirror, or the back of your front door. When you place your chart where you can see it without effort, you are changing your environment in a way that will increase your chances of engaging in the desired behavior.

Finally, the monitoring chart serves as a visual reinforcement or reward. By watching your progress on the chart, you feel proud and confident, and you will be more likely to continue the behavior.

Arrange Your World for Success

Making changes in your environment, or "arranging your world for success," is surprisingly simple, and it can have immediate positive effects on your behavior. For example, at a recent dinner with colleagues and friends, the topic turned to unhealthy habits. One dinner guest described her habit of adding extra salt to her food and asked for help with decreasing her salt intake. As the token psychologists at the table, we told her we would help her decrease the chance of ingesting additional salt with her meal right at that moment. All the other guests were waiting for some sort of hocus-pocus.

Instead, we scanned the dinner table (evaluated her environment). We noticed the salt shaker was within arm's length of the woman, so we simply moved it to the opposite end of the table. We proclaimed with great satisfaction that this gesture had significantly decreased her chances of using excess salt during the meal. Everyone thought this was silly, but guess what? The woman did not use extra salt for the rest of the meal, even though she said she normally would have. The point is that changing your environment can have immediate and powerful effects on your behavior.

Arranging the world around you means doing things that will increase the odds of your being successful with changing your target behavior. No one can be successful 100 percent of the time. Life will always throw challenges your way. You may be going along nicely with an exercise program and then get sick and be unable to exercise for a week. You may be sticking with a healthy diet and then the holidays roll around. You may have out-of-town guests to entertain. The weather might be bad, the car can break down, your boss can ask you to stay late at work, or the kids can get sick—the list goes on and on. There are some things you simply can't control. This is why we want you to take charge of the things you can control in order to succeed.

Arranging your world means changing your immediate surroundings to increase the chances of a healthy behavior, such as a proper diet or exercise, or to decrease the chance of an unhealthy behavior, such as smoking. If you want to eat low-calorie foods but you have a pantry stuffed with cookies and chips, the chances of eating the low-calorie foods are slim. However, if you want to eat low-calorie fat foods and your pantry contains nothing but low-calorie foods, you're much more likely to eat them. Unfortunately, many people fail to arrange their environments to promote positive change. They simply don't recognize the power of the environment.

The challenge is to make your environment support your desired target behavior so that it becomes easy to do, but how do you do this? Try this simple exercise.

If you want to exercise every morning, think about how to modify your environment to increase your chances of success. Go ahead and list your ideas

Changes I Can Make to My World That Will Promote Morning Exercise

1._____

2._____

3._____

4._____

5._____

6._____

Here are some of the suggestions we came up with. You may have similar ideas, or you might have thought of others not on our list.

> Set the alarm clock to include the amount of time it takes to get ready + travel time + exercise time.
> Before going to bed, lay out your exercise clothes where you will see them immediately upon rising.
> The night before, prepare any food or drink you plan to have before exercising.
> Inform others (family, friends, your dog) that you *will* (not that you *plan* to) exercise in the morning.

In an ideal world, someone would come to your bedroom each morning, wake you, dress you, feed you, take you to your exercise location, and exercise with you. Just think, what would

JOSHUA KLAPOW, SHERI PRUITT

be the chances of not exercising under these circumstances? Because most of us cannot afford this kind of assistance, we must try to get as close to it as possible. If you do the four things listed above, but still don't exercise, it will be due to either an emergency or illness, or because you make the choice not to exercise.

Arranging your world for success is all about taking control of your surroundings in small but powerful ways. If you can arrange the world around you to support the behavioral change you want to make, you will find that making and sticking with changes gets easier and easier. List below a health behavior that you want to change other than exercise, such as eat healthy food, quit smoking, get more sleep, or remember to take your medication. Then, list the things you can do to set yourself up for success. With a little thought you can be successful in creating an environment that supports your healthy changes. Remember, make it as easy as possible to do your target behavior.

Behavior I want to change: _____

Ways I can arrange my world to support this change

1._____

2._____

3._____

4._____

5._____

6._____

7._____

ACTION TIP

Getting over Gym Phobia

Going to a gym or health club can be a little intimidating, so here are some tips to help you ease into the gym experience. Find a gym or club that is close to your home or work—the closer, the more likely you are to go. Then take a tour and ask as many questions as you want before you join. Make sure it's the right gym for you. Take advantage of free personal training or use of a trainer for a short time; you'll get familiar with the equipment and develop a workout routine. Finally, if you're feeling a little self-conscious, train at off-peak hours when the gym is less crowded. Remember, every person in the gym was unsure of himself in the beginning. Everyone there is trying to improve. The longer you stick with it, the more comfortable it will become.

Recruit a Support Team

Ultimately, the changes you make to your lifestyle are your responsibility; they are under your control and will primarily benefit you. However, your family, friends, co-workers, and others can play a big role in your success (Wing & Jeffery, 1999). The people in your life can be powerful motivators, strong reinforcers, and unfortunately sometimes the major barriers to making lifestyle changes. Family, friends, and co-workers are a part of your environment. As we discussed in the section on arranging your world for success, the people in your life can either facilitate lifestyle change or slow it down.

Now that you know this, work to maximize the positive influence of others. The key is to take charge and set up a team of supporters who will be encouraging and work with you. Most often, people leave the influence of those around them up to chance. They try to make changes on their own, and are either pleasantly surprised when friends and family offer encouragement and support, or frustrated when they seem uninterested or act as obstacles to change. If you are going to make the effort to change your lifestyle and become healthier, why leave such a potentially powerful influence to chance? Let's take a look at what you can do to "rally the troops."

Think of those around you as an "army" of support. This may sound a bit self-centered. After all, you're not paying for their help the way you would professionals, such as trainers, coaches, or counselors. In reality, however, family, friends, co-workers, and even total strangers often are willing to help you make changes to improve your health without expecting anything in return. Why? We want to think that most people are just naturally eager to help one another.

If you think about this idea from a slightly more skeptical, yet scientific, perspective, it does make sense. Helping others can be a rewarding experience that is reinforced by the feelings it produces. For many people, knowing their actions have helped someone lose weight, stop smoking, become more physically fit, overcome an addiction, or reduce stress produces feelings of satisfaction, contentment, and even empowerment. Simply put, it just feels good to help others.

The people who agree to help you can be placed into two categories: change partners and supporters. Both are good, and both can help. Let's take a look at what each has to offer.

Change Partners. Change partners are people similar to you; they are also trying to make a lifestyle change. You can partner with them in your mutual endeavors. The advantage of being change partners is that both partners will have the satisfaction of helping someone else and the support they need for changing their own behaviors.

Supporters. Although supporters are not necessarily making changes themselves, they have agreed to support you and "be there" for you throughout the process. They may already have undergone the changes you are trying to make, or they may simply care about you enough to support your attempt to change your lifestyle.

Ideally, you will find a number of partners and supporters, but don't worry if you can't assemble an all-star team right away. Having a few dedicated people on your side is better than having either no one or a lot of people who aren't really committed to your goals. Now that you know other people can benefit from helping you, here is what you can do:

> ➢ Decide what kind of support will be most helpful.
> ➢ See what kind of support and providers are available.
> ➢ Go out and ask for the exact support you need.

Finding a Change Partner. Let's start with change partners. Where and how do you find them? Potential change partners are all around you— you simply haven't looked for them (or, maybe you think you don't need support—think again!). A change partner can be your spouse or significant other, a friend, a parent, or another relative. Sometimes a potential partner will have already embarked on a lifestyle change and be struggling. In this case, the opportunity to get help and support (from you) will be most welcome. Other potential partners might be well on their way to making changes of their own and will share their experiences to bring you up to speed.

Consider your family and friends. Who among them is trying to change their lifestyle? Who is trying to exercise, diet, quit smoking, or make some other change? You probably never really looked at them as potential partners. Besides family, think about where you spend the majority of your time; who at your school or work is trying to make lifestyle changes? Does that person know you want to make a change, too? Again, we'd bet that you have never talked directly with this person and suggested a team approach. Becoming change partners can help both of you succeed. The following are places where you might consider looking for a partner:

➢ Home.
➢ Work.
➢ School.
➢ Religious congregations.
➢ Social gatherings (parks, bookstores, malls, fitness facilities).
➢ Virtual communities (reputable health and fitness Web sites with chat rooms or partner programs).

Who would make a good change partner? Should you simply choose anyone making a lifestyle change that is willing to partner with you? Although you don't have to be too fussy, you should follow these general guidelines:

➢ Choose someone who is as committed to changing health behaviors as you are.
➢ Choose a partner who has similar, but not necessarily identical, goals.
➢ Choose a person whose daily schedule will allow him to work with you in making changes; for example, working out together, shopping for groceries together, eating together, or talking to one another regularly about the progress you are both making.

List three or more potential change partners. If you don't know their names, just describe them (for example, the woman you see walking in the park every morning).

1. _____

2. _____

3. _____

4. _____

5. _____

Finding a Supporter. Supporters are often easier to find than change partners, and you'll have a wider selection of people from which to choose, because they don't personally have to make lifestyle changes in order to qualify. Finding supporters also starts with looking at the people around you. Your immediate family and friends are important potential supporters. The difference between a supportive spouse or significant other and someone who has little interest in your lifestyle changes can really influence your success.

One of the best places to start looking for supporters is at home. Talk with the people closest to you. Be straightforward. Tell them about your goals, your concerns and fears, and why you need them to be there for you. Recruit them to support your new behavior. Let them know that supporting you won't require a lot of effort on their part but that their support is critical to your success. Remember, most people want to be helpful, particularly when it doesn't require much work. Supporters who live with you may be affected by your lifestyle changes more than those who don't. The changes you make in the foods you eat, the way you spend your time on a daily basis—such as going to the gym, walking in the park, going to bed earlier, practicing meditation, not going to bars, and not frequenting fast-food establishments—may have a significant effect on the people you're with the most. In that case, it can be immensely helpful to have supporters who are willing to become partners.

Having other people around you who are doing the things you want to stop doing will definitely create a challenge. Why? Think about the SMART skill: "Arrange Your World for Success." If you plan to stop eating high-fat foods, and your spouse, children, or the other people you live with keep these foods in abundance in the house, you are living in an environment that is less conducive to a low-fat diet. The same applies to things such as smoking, not exercising, excessive drinking, and poor sleep habits. Basically, if someone else is living an unhealthy lifestyle in your environment it will probably decrease your chances of success in making healthy changes.

Does this mean you will fail? No. Does it mean you will have more obstacles to overcome? Yes.

Therefore, you may need to ask family and friends to make some changes in their own lifestyles in order to support you. Although everyone might not be willing, you may be pleasantly surprised to find that they will readily make the small changes you ask of them if they see the changes are beneficial. This might include not smoking around you, being a bit more flexible with daily schedules so you have time to exercise, or changing some of the social activities you participate in together.

Your success is one of the greatest rewards you can give your family and friends. If they see that their "sacrifices" are helping you become a healthier person, they are more likely to stick with you and the changes you have asked them to make. Let's put it this way: It's pretty hard to justify asking your family to give you time to exercise and not to eat junk food around you if they see you lying on the couch, watching television, and eating a big bag of chips!

Just how "healthy" do your supporters need to be? As a general rule, the more time you spend with a potential supporter on a daily basis, the more important it is for their health habits to be in line with your goals. If your Auntie Mae lives a thousand miles away but has agreed to talk with you any time you want or need to, she probably doesn't need to change her own eating or exercise habits in order to support you. However, your spouse, children, or co-workers, with whom you spend the majority of your time, will be a lot more helpful if their own lifestyle habits are in line with your goals.

The other advantage in having supporters whose lifestyles are consistent with your goals is that they are likely to be more sincere and enthusiastic in their support. It's more difficult for someone who eats poorly, doesn't exercise, and smokes to say with sincerity that they believe in the changes you are trying to make and understand their importance. This doesn't mean that someone with poor lifestyle habits isn't capable of caring about you and the changes you are trying to make; it simply means they may be less committed to your goals.

ACTION TIP

Stop Nagging

It's frustrating. You try to eat a low-fat diet and exercise, but your spouse isn't motivated to do the same. When it comes to changing health habits, spouses don't always see eye to eye. Although encouraging a spouse or loved one to take the steps they need for better health is important, encouragement alone may not always work. Instead, help your spouse by asking specific "action questions."

Start by asking what you can do to help your spouse to make the desired changes. Ask how important it is to your spouse to be healthy. You can also ask if more information would be helpful, such as figuring out the best eating plan or learning more about intensity and frequency of exercise. If your spouse knows what to do, ask if you can help to create a plan for getting started. Encouragement is important, but action questions can really get the ball rolling.

In general, a supporter should be a person who:

➢ Cares about your health and well-being.
➢ Is willing to make small sacrifices to help you achieve your goals.
➢ Spends a significant amount of time with you on a daily basis.
➢ Has earned your respect and appreciation.

List three or more people who could be your supporters.

1. _____

2. _____

3. _____

4. _____

5. _____

What specific support will you ask for?

1. _____

2. _____

3. _____

4. _____

5. _____

Can I Go It Alone? If recruiting a support team doesn't appeal to you, or if you don't have anyone in your life right now, you may be wondering whether you can make lifestyle changes on your own. Remember, the SMART skills described in this book are designed to help you be successful in changing your lifestyle. The more skills you can use, the more likely you will have success. This doesn't mean you will fail if you don't have a support team. Many people have been able to make lifestyle changes without support. However, years of research show that the right kind of support is helpful. Don't give up if you can't rally a team, and don't spend the next 6 months waiting to start changing your behavior until you find the perfect supporters. Spend a few weeks looking for people who can work with you. Then, whether you have assembled a team or not, use the other SMART skills and move forward.

Continue to look for partners and supporters as you embark on your lifestyle changes. You may find that friends, family, and co-workers will notice and encourage you. You may also find it easier to approach people and request their support. Finally, you will probably start to encounter people who are potential partners or supporters as you discover new places associated with your lifestyle changes; for example, groups, parks, workout facilities, new restaurants, new Web sites, even new sections of the grocery store. Finding the right support team may take some time, so start making lifestyle changes and search for team members along the way.

Treat Yourself

One of the most basic principles of behavioral science is that rewarded behaviors are more likely to be repeated (Skinner, 1953). This principle is referred to as reinforcement, and it affects everyone—pets, children, and adults. We are using "treat" as a reward or reinforcement. Understanding how reinforcement works will help you harness its power to make changes in your behavior.

Positive reinforcement occurs when a behavior is followed by an event that increases the chances that the behavior will be repeated. This process can take many forms. For example, positive reinforcement could include receiving money for a job well done, getting a compliment from a friend after you've changed your diet, or giving your child some screen time for cleaning her room. In each case, the chance of the particular behavior (doing a good job, diet change, and room cleaning) being repeated is likely to be improved because it is associated with a pleasant event. Positive reinforcement is a great strategy for creating new behaviors.

With negative reinforcement, the chance that a behavior will be repeated is increased by removing something that is unpleasant. For example, if you have a headache and find that you can escape this unpleasant feeling by taking an aspirin, the behavior of taking the aspirin is likely to be repeated the next time you have a headache.

Keep in mind that the terms "positive" and "negative" don't necessarily refer to "good" and "bad." Negative reinforcement is not the same thing as punishment. If used properly, both types of reinforcement can help you continue performing your desired behaviors.

Reinforcement can take a variety of forms. All kinds of treats—money, verbal praise, telling yourself "great job," applause, or gold stars on a monitoring chart—can increase your chance of repeating a desired behavior. What works best? That's the tricky part, and it's an individual thing. What might be a powerful treat for one person might not be for someone else.

Chances are you already know what kinds of rewards are likely to increase your chances of success in changing your behavior. Here are some broad categories.

Circle the ones that might work for you that you could get frequently and immediately:

➢ Monetary rewards (cash placed in a jar).
➢ Internal rewards (saying to yourself, "great job!").
➢ Non-monetary rewards (a phone call with a friend, a "star" or "points" on your chart).
➢ Social rewards (praise from friends and family).
➢ Activity rewards (taking a break, going out for some fresh air).
➢ Physiological rewards (pleasant sights, sounds, tastes, and smells).
➢ Psychological rewards (recognizing feelings of happiness, contentment, and satisfaction).

Notice that tasty treats are not on the list of rewards. Why do we get into so much trouble with sweets, salty snacks, and other junk food? Food has the potential to be a powerful physiologic and psychological reward—it's a reinforcer that satisfies both our bodies and our minds. As an example, think about eating ice cream, which has a built-in reward system for most people. You purchase the ice cream and put some in your mouth. It's cool, refreshing, sweet, and creamy. Your taste buds come alive, and your visual, olfactory, and gustatory senses are stimulated. You smile. You're happy. Thus your ice cream eating behavior has been rewarded. What happens next? You take another bite, and another, and every bite you take gives you both physiologic and psychological rewards. This is the reason that tasty food rewards are not a great idea: too powerful, too available, and too easily over-consumed.

Once you have figured out what rewards are important for you, when should you give them to yourself? Again, we know from behavioral science that new behaviors need to be rewarded frequently and immediately in order to become established. The goal is to create a permanent habit over time.

Developing a new habit means rewarding the new behavior--immediately and over and over again--until it becomes part of your routine. Once it becomes a habit, you can back off the rewards a bit. With time, you may find that the behavior itself has rewarding properties; for example, feelings of accomplishment and satisfaction. This frees you from having to reward the behavior each and every time. However, ongoing occasional rewards will keep the new behavior going strong. As silly as it sounds, the simple treat of telling yourself "I did it!" or "good work!" has been proven to work.

ACTION TIP

Effective Treats

Use these strategies to maximize the Principle of Reinforcement

- ➤ Decide on the reward before you start to make changes in your behavior.
- ➤ Be intentional about treating yourself.
- ➤ Determine exactly when and how often you will treat yourself.
- ➤ Consider including your rewards on your monitoring chart and post it where you'll see it every day and know your progress and what you're working toward.
- ➤ Make sure that your rewards occur after every behavior in the beginning. For example, reward yourself after every exercise session or every meal that you eat that is within your calorie range.
- ➤ Use small, frequent treats, such as a brief chat with a friend on the phone or taking the time to watch the sunset. These are good rewards. Think of them as such. Plan to treat yourself with something that is immediate and gives you pleasure.

Treat Yourself Checklist Exercise

Fill in the blanks to create your reward schedule:

I will give myself _____ (reward) as a treat for _____ (health behavior).

I will give myself _____ (reward) on the following schedule: _____ _____ (how often you will give yourself the reward).

In addition to giving myself _____ (reward), if I complete _____ (number of days, weeks, or months) of _____ (health behavior), I will give myself a special bonus treat of _____ (choose a bonus reward such as a movie, a manicure, or new walking shoes).

Remember, a behavior that is rewarded, or "treated," is likely to be repeated. If you consistently reward your exercise, diet, and non-smoking behaviors in the beginning, over time you will find that these healthy behaviors have become rewarding on their own, and the need for continued treats will slowly fade.

5

Stay on Track—Avoid Behavioral Drift

Now that you have learned the SMART skills, you can use them in combination with accurate information and your internal motivation to be successful in making lasting lifestyle changes. However, being successful does not mean being perfect. No matter how dedicated and committed you are, there will be periodic setbacks, but why? First, life throws up all kinds of obstacles to change—illness, injury, vacation, and work and home responsibilities. We interact with an environment that is constantly changing. Second, you are basically taking old behaviors and replacing them with new ones. The key word here is "new." The behaviors are not yet learned habits, and you will have a tendency to slip back into your old patterns.

Behavioral Drift

We call slipping back into old patterns *behavioral drift*. It refers to the tendency to go back to old behavioral patterns when you are first making changes (see relapse prevention; Marlatt & George, 1984). Everyone is affected by behavioral drift. It is not a matter of *if* it will happen, but *when* it will happen. We are all creatures of habit— and habits are strong, powerful things. When you begin to make changes in your lifestyle, there will be a strong pull toward your old habits. Behavioral drift affects everyone all the time. It's incredibly common, yet many people wonder why they seem to shift gradually back to their old ways just when they think they are doing a good at job at changing them. Behavioral drift always seems to sneak up on people, grab them, and pull them back to their old patterns of behavior. No one ever warns us about behavioral drift. Well, consider this a warning.

Don't worry, though. Knowing that behavioral drift exists is the most important part of managing it. Now, let's discuss how to deal with it.

Don't Let the Drift Catch You. Now that you have read up to this point, you actually have everything you need to deal with the dreaded behavioral drift. Nothing in this section is new, except for an understanding of the drift itself. Here's a quick preview of how the skills you've learned can help:

> Monitoring your progress and using the other SMART skills will help you recognize the early stages of drift.
> Your understanding of motivation, rewards, and environmental barriers will enable you to find the cause of the drift.
> Your ability to recruit a support team and set achievable goals will help you modify any drift that does occur.

You see, once you have the tools to defeat it, the drift process is not quite so scary.

Dealing with behavioral drift involves three key actions:

1. Anticipating the causes of the drift.
2. Having a plan to deal with the drift.
3. Catching the drift as early as possible.

JOSHUA KLAPOW, SHERI PRUITT

ACTION TIP

Navigating the Grocery Aisles

Shopping for groceries can be tough when you're trying to eat healthier foods. How do you resist buying the high-calorie items that are not good for you? You're going to face temptations, but these simple tips will help:

➤ Write out your grocery list ahead of time. Not having a list puts you at risk of buying things that don't meet your goals. Check off each item as you shop.

➤ Avoid going up and down each aisle. Use your list to navigate past the cookies, chips, and other tempting items. Try shopping the perimeter of the store.

➤ Go shopping with a buddy, so you can focus on conversation rather than temptation.

➤ Reward yourself for sticking with your grocery list by purchasing one small treat for yourself such as a special tea, coffee, or sparkling water.

Anticipating the Causes of the Drift. You have already done the most important part—you have learned that behavioral drift can and will occur. Now, make a list of the situations that are likely to cause you to back-slide from your new lifestyle behaviors. This "What If" list will help you target situations that are likely to lead to behavioral drift. The details of this list will be different for each behavior, but the process and general topics are the same. Here are some common examples:

➤ What if the weather is bad and I can't exercise outside?

➤ What if we go out to dinner and they don't have the foods on my eating plan?

➤ What if we are traveling and I can't get to bed at a reasonable hour?

➤ What if I go to a bar and someone offers me a cigarette?

➤ What if my schedule changes and I can't do my relaxation exercises in the morning before work?

➤ What if my motivation levels decrease?

➤ What if the rewards I am using no longer work?

➤ What if I am sick or injured and unable to exercise, prepare certain meals, or take my scheduled medications?

➤ What if my change partner is no longer available?

➤ What if my supporters aren't giving me the support I need?

List three or more "What If" scenarios that might affect your success in achieving your new lifestyle goals.

1. _____

2. _____

3. _____

4. _____

These situations will not necessarily cause behavioral drift, but they are good warning signs. Therefore, the longer the list, the more helpful it will be. Leave no stone unturned. If you can anticipate it, you can plan for it—and if you can plan for it, you will know how to deal with it.

A Plan for Getting Back on Track

1. Answering the "What Ifs"

    To develop your plan for dealing with behavioral drift, you need to come up with one or more answers for each of your "What If" scenarios. These situations do not perfectly predict that drift will occur, but if it does, you will be able to remedy the problem. Similarly, if you find yourself drifting back into your old habits, you can use the "What If" list to figure out the possible cause. Here are some feasible answers and plans for action to "What If" questions:

What if I can't exercise outdoors because the weather is bad?
Even if I can't walk outside, I can walk indoors at the local mall, or I can march in place while watching television.

What if I can't do my normal exercise routine because I will be out of town?
Even if I am out of town, I can call ahead and see if there are similar workout facilities where I will be staying, or I can walk inside or outside for 15 minutes.

What if my motivation level seems to be slipping?
Even if my motivation dips, I can challenge myself by answering the following questions honestly:

> ➤ What are the benefits of this new behavior?
> ➤ How important is it to improve my health?
> ➤ What is really important to me?
> ➤ What am I doing right now instead of the new behavior?
> ➤ Are the reasons for NOT doing it more important than bettering my health?

2.   Your Drift Partner

In addition to answering the "What Ifs," your supporters can help you manage behavioral drift. Designate one person on your support team to be your drift partner. Ask this person's permission to call and talk when you first notice the signs of drift. Your drift partner will encourage you to get back on track immediately and remind you of your goals and what's important to you.

3.   The Three-Day Rule

Now that you're armed with a plan for dealing with situations that can cause drift, you are ready to set up your "Drift Radar." Actually, you already have—your monitoring chart is the best way to alert you when you begin to drift. The rule of thumb for catching drift is to let the monitoring chart speak for itself. Don't guess at whether or not, and to what extent, you have done a new behavior; the monitoring chart will serve as your radar screen.

Monitoring is "black and white." By marking down your new health-related behaviors (exercise, dietary intake, taking medication, or number of days of non-smoking), you will know whether or not you have practiced your target behavior. If the behavior seems to slip off the radar screen for a period of time, a red flag should be raised, and you will need to look at your "What If" list to see what's going on and what needs to be done.

As a general guideline, you are starting to drift if you have gone more than 3 days without practicing your new behavior. There may be good reasons why you haven't practiced the behavior, but that is not the point. In the early stages of lifestyle change, every day that a new behavior isn't practiced is another lost day of habit development. Even if you have good reasons for failing to practice your new behavior, simply not doing it will contribute to the drift. Look at your monitoring chart every day and be prepared. Catch drift early, have a plan and do an immediate course correction.

Putting Everything into Perspective

Finally, put all of this information into perspective. If your goal is to eat a healthier diet, exercise regularly, practice relaxation exercises, get adequate sleep, or wear your seat belt every time you drive for the rest of your life, then missing 2 or 3 days of your new behavior is not the end of the world. The critical point is that you need to catch behavioral drift as soon as you see it, implement your plan, and get back on track. If you don't take the time to deal with drift, 2–3 days may turn into 2–3 weeks, months, or years. Anticipating the drift, knowing what situations can cause it, and having a plan to deal with it will keep you on the right track.

Ultimately it comes down to this: You are in control of your health, and you have the tools and techniques to make lifestyle changes. This is not magic. It's not a mystery. You can change any lifestyle behavior you want to and ultimately become a healthier person.

ACTION TIP

Accepting Negative Emotions

You try so hard to lose weight, exercise, or quit smoking. Then you have a setback, and with it comes guilt, self-doubt, and fading confidence. The trick is to accept these negative thoughts as part of the normal process of the ups and downs of lifestyle change. When you have a setback, take a minute to examine what you're thinking, the emotions you're experiencing, and the feelings you're having in the moment. Let these negative thoughts float from your mind. Visualize them gently leaving your head. You don't need to fight them or change them. These are simply thoughts in your mind that you have created. Your thoughts don't direct your actions. You choose what to do. You always have the power to behave in line with your goals and values.

6

The Chart: Your All-in-One Behavior Change Tool

The Chart
The What, The Want, and The How

My health behavior is: _____(be specific)

I will practice my behavior_____days per week.

My short-term goal is _____.

My long-term goal is _____.

I will give myself _____(treat)
on the following schedule:
_____(how often).

In addition to giving myself _____, when I
complete _____ (number of days, weeks, or months),
I will give myself a bonus treat of _____.

SUN	MON	TUE	WED	THU	FRI	SAT

Everything you have read so far can be condensed into this monitoring chart, which can be used to track your healthy changes. The only catch is that you must first have a general understanding of the previous material in the book. Once you understand the three necessary components: The What, The Want, and The How, this chart will help you change your target behaviors.

We call this tool simply "The Chart," because on one level that is all that it is, a piece of paper. However, The Chart is also a lifestyle-change tool that contains the essential components necessary for changing behavior.

The What

The Chart shows you what to do on a daily basis, how much you are supposed to do, and how frequently you should do it.

The Want

The Chart allows you to see your lifestyle change achievements on a daily, weekly, and monthly basis. Seeing your progress in black and white is a terrific reminder of your success. Success feels good, and confidence strengthens your motivation to keep going. You can see your progress, that you have the ability to change, and that you're doing what you set out to do.

The How

The Chart helps you accomplish all of the SMART behavior change skills discussed in this book.

Here's how it works:

Set a Goal:

The Chart allows you to specify your target behaviors. It outlines what, when, and for how long you will do your target behavior-the one you're confident that you can achieve.

Monitor Your Progress:

The Chart allows you to keep track of your health-related behaviors and the progress toward your goal. It holds you accountable to yourself and takes the guess work out of what you're doing.

Arrange Your World for Success:

The Chart is a visual reminder--if posted where you can easily see it--that will cue you to do the behaviors that are important to you.

Recruit a Support Team:

The Chart allows you to show others your specific lifestyle goals and recruit their support in your change effort.

Treat Yourself:

If you use visual rewards, such as gold stars or points that you mark on a daily basis, using The Chart becomes the reward. It also allows you to see the special bonus rewards you will give yourself after you have practiced healthy target behaviors over a period of time.

This simple piece of paper can be a huge help when you are trying to make lifestyle changes. Making a chart can be as easy as grabbing a calendar and writing down your target behaviors, short- and long-term goals, and rewards. You can get more elaborate and design a chart on your computer, but more complicated charts are not necessarily better. In fact, the real key to The Chart's helpfulness and usefulness is your ability to look at it every day and maintain it without a lot of effort. A simple calendar posted on your refrigerator will be much more effective than a complex, custom-designed chart that sits in a drawer or in a stack of papers or in an app on your phone that you don't open. So keep your chart simple, and put it on your refrigerator door today. Think of The Chart as your secret weapon. No one would ever suspect that such a simple thing could give you the edge in making successful lifestyle changes.

PART 2

Your Game Plan

You now have all the ingredients to make *any* change in *any* lifestyle behavior you want. That's a pretty powerful concept, but one that can also be a bit overwhelming. The following chapters will help you put the ideas in this book into specific actions.

This section contains specific *game plans* for change. We've chosen four common issues that many people struggle with: sticking with an eating plan or exercise program, getting better sleep, and remembering to take medication. These game plans offer unique tips that are suited for these particular health behaviors, and they can help you jump start your progress. Remember, you can use the same SMART skills to change any other lifestyle behavior that is getting in the way of your good health.

7

My Diet Game Plan

The What—Important Information about Your Diet

The average American's diet is not great. Just take a look at these figures from a study published in the Journal of Food Composition and Analysis:

> ➤ Sweets and desserts, soft drinks, and alcoholic beverages make up almost 25 percent of all calories consumed by Americans.
> ➤ Salty snacks and fruit-flavored drinks comprise 5 percent of the calories consumed by Americans.
> ➤ Healthy foods, such as vegetables and fruit, make up only 10 percent of the caloric intake in the U.S. diet.
> ➤ A large proportion of Americans are undernourished in terms of vitamins and minerals, even though they eat a lot of food.

A key conclusion from this study is that people shouldn't necessarily be eating less, they should be eating differently. Most of us eat too many foods that are high in saturated fat and added sugar and these foods have relatively more calories than other foods. Here are some simple tips from the U.S. Department of Agriculture and the Choose My Plate program to eat a healthier diet. (For more information see http://www.choosemyplate.gov).

➤ Include food and drink choices from all five food groups: fruits, vegetables, grains, protein foods, and dairy to get essential nutrients.
➤ Choose foods and drinks that are low in saturated fat, sodium, and added sugars.
➤ Read the Nutrition Facts labels, check the serving size, and look at the list of ingredients.
➤ Eat the right amount of calories for you based on your age, sex, height, weight, and level of physical activity.
➤ Make half your plate fruits and vegetables.
➤ Focus on whole fruits.
➤ Vary the types of vegetables.
➤ Make half your grains whole grains.
➤ Eat lower fat and fat-free dairy.
➤ Vary your protein choices.

ACTION TIP

Control Your Snacking Habits

Are you a snacker? Snacking is a habit for many people. It has little to do with hunger, and can keep you from reaching your health goals. Here are some tips to help you curb your snacking habit:

➤ Keep a food diary for 1 week. As you record what you eat, write down what you were doing at the time and whether or not you were actually hungry. This will help you identify your snacking pattern. For example, you may tend to snack while watching television.
➤ Manage situations where you tend to snack by substituting other activities that make it hard to snack. Try playing with your kids or pets, or exercise while you watch television.

Knowing your snacking patterns and having actions to prevent them will help improve your eating habits.

The Want—Are You Motivated to Change Your Eating Habits?

This is the time to be honest about what you really want to do about your eating habits. The simple question is: How important is it to you to change? Are you motivated to do things differently? If your answer to this question is "no, I'm not at all motivated to change" you will not likely be able to change your eating behavior and this is probably not a good time for you to try to do something about your diet. You may want to tackle your eating habits at another time, or you could review the exercises in Chapter 3 to tap into your internal motivation to be healthier. Either way, the principles and SMART skills outlined in this book will still be available when you feel more confident that you can change.

If your answer to this question is "yes" I want to change my eating habits—great! Some degree of motivation is necessary to change behavior and to keep it going over the long term. You have to have some level of desire to make changes, recognize your reasons for changing, and appreciate that you need to do things differently with your eating in order to be successful.

Let's examine more closely the degree to which you're motivated to change your eating habits. Rate your level of motivation on the scale below.

| 1 | 2 | 3 | 4 | 5 | 6 | 7 | 8 | 9 | 10 |

Not motivated   Completely motivated

If your degree of motivation is less than 3, go back to Chapter 3 and use the motivation-boosting strategies. It's important to find your own reasons for changing your eating patterns. Eating a healthy diet needs to be important to you personally in order for you to be motivated to change. If you rated your motivation as 4 or greater, you're ready to get started. Remember, you don't have to be a "10"—completely motivated. If you rate yourself at mid-point on the scale, you have enough motivation to start changing your eating habits. As we've said before, motivation typically fluctuates over time. Whenever you feel your motivation fading, go back and use the boosters in Chapter 3.

The How—SMART Skills That Can Change Your Eating Habits

SMART skills are the key to changing habits and routines. You read about them earlier, but now let's make them specific to eating. Read through the examples below to see what you can use to help you start your new eating habits.

Set a Goal. Goals for improving eating habits are as numerous and individual as the people who want to change their diets. However, some eating goals pop up more frequently than others, and they have several common themes. We often get comments such as: "I want to consume fewer calories," "My goal is to eat less fast food," or "My goal is to cut sweets, sodas, and desserts out of my diet."

These are great ideas, but they are too general. Remember, setting a goal requires you to be specific—the more specific, observable, and measurable the goal, the more likely you are to succeed. You need to identify a behavior that is observable and that can be measured. You need to be sure that it is a goal you can achieve—don't set yourself up for failure. How could you make the goal, "I want to consume fewer calories" specific, observable, and measurable?

Write your answers below:

General goal: "I want to consume fewer calories."

Make it specific: _____
_____.

How could you observe it? _____
_____.

How could you measure it? _____
_____.

We came up with a specific goal of "eat 1,600 calories per day." This is observable, because you can see yourself putting food portions containing a certain number of calories into your mouth. Also, calories can be counted or measured. Calorie content can be found in books or on the Internet, and labels on most foods identify the number of calories in a serving (be sure to double check the number of servings in a package or a container—often there are more than one).

How can you make the general goal "I want to eat less fast food," specific, observable, and measurable?

Make it specific: _____
_____.
How could you observe it? _____
_____.
How could you measure it? _____
_____.

Monitor Your Progress. Monitoring what you eat and reducing your caloric intake takes a bit of effort. It's important to keep track of the calories in everything you eat and drink during the day. So, you need to keep your monitoring chart close by, because you probably eat at home, work, and in restaurants or fast food places. Some people use a phone app for this because a phone is always handy. Others make multiple copies of the monitoring chart (see Chapter 6) and keep it in a pocket, briefcase, or handbag. Make sure that whatever approach you use for monitoring works for you and that your monitoring method is always within easy reach. You don't want to rely on your memory. That won't work.

ACTION TIP

Managing Fast Food Temptations

In today's fast-paced lifestyle, fast food is a major convenience. But it can quickly become a very unhealthy habit. If you're on a diet, you know how hard it is to resist visiting your favorite fast food restaurants. If fast food is your weakness, try these tips:

➤ Bring your lunch to work, and plan dinners at home so you aren't tempted to eat out.
➤ If your favorite fast food restaurant is on your daily commute, change your route or place a sticky note on your dashboard that says, "No Fast Food."
➤ Avoid getting fast food for your kids. Your family will benefit from healthier meals.
➤ Choose a special reward (not food related) for you and your family for each day you skip fast food.

Before you know it, fast food will become less tempting, and you'll reach your health goals more quickly.

Keeping track of fast foods and desserts may be somewhat easier. If you set a goal of limiting fast food meals to one per week, you could use your monitoring chart to keep track of this behavior. Be sure to post the chart in a visible place, so you are reminded of your goal and your weekly progress. Similarly, if you are trying to decrease the number of desserts and sugary snacks in your diet, the monitoring chart or a calendar on the wall will work perfectly.

Arrange Your World for Success. The environment around you is incredibly powerful in pulling behavior from you. You can harness this power to pull the "right" behaviors and help you meet your eating goals. The idea is to set up the world around you so that you are successful in changing your eating habits. If you don't have high-calorie foods in your environment, you won't be able to eat them. If you don't bring fast food into your world, you won't eat it. These strategies make perfect sense when you think about making the world around you support your efforts for successful eating.

Use these strategies to eat the foods that help you meet your goals:

➤ Remove all high-calorie foods from your kitchen and pantry.
➤ If you must have special snacks for your children, keep them in a place where you can't see them, keep them out of easy reach, and have an alternative available for you.

> ➤ "Arranging" begins at the grocery store. Only bring home food that will help you meet your goals.
> ➤ Have healthy snacks visible and readily available so you can get to them easily if you feel tempted to eat a high- calorie food.
> ➤ Post a reminder to yourself on the refrigerator door about your eating goals. Your monitoring chart could serve this purpose.
> ➤ Pack a healthy lunch the night before so that it's ready to take to work with you in the morning.

Recruit a Support Team. Research shows that this SMART skill is highly effective—having support from others will definitely help you stick with any diet and successfully change your eating habits. The problem is that not everyone is likely to be aware of your goal, so you may not automatically get the support you need. Tell people you are making changes in your eating habits, but also tell them exactly what they can do to help you. Here are some simple, useful strategies for getting support:

> ➤ Let your family and friends know you are trying to change your eating habits and stick with a healthier diet;
> ➤ Talk with them about how challenging this is for you, and let them know their help is critical for your success.

There are many ways other people can support your efforts, some of which may be more practical and feasible than others:

> ➤ Ask them if they would like to join you in changing eating habits.
> ➤ Ask them to periodically give you verbal encouragement and praise for sticking with your plan.
> ➤ Ask them to call and leave encouraging messages.
> ➤ Ask if they will send you supportive e-mails or text messages.
> ➤ Let your spouse or significant other know exactly what help you need to stick with your diet, such as not eating dessert in front of you or not offering you foods that don't meet your goals.

Treat Yourself. A new diet or any other change in your eating habits that is painful or depriving simply will not work for the long term. You need some ongoing benefit or reward from your diet to keep you going over time. What can you do to treat yourself? If your goal is to lose 20 pounds by eating a healthier diet, and you believe your reward will be the lost weight, you are simply setting yourself up for failure. Why? You will fail because you will not lose 20 pounds in the first week—you may not even lose 2 pounds!

What will keep you going? What treat or reward will get you through the first day of the diet and on to the second? How will you treat yourself after week one so you can continue on to week two? If you build treats into your eating plan such that a treat follows every meal, snack or drink that is in line with your goals, you will be more likely to stick with these changes and ultimately reach your long term goal. Does treating yourself mean a banana split or a pizza at the end of the week? Absolutely not. Here are some ideas about how you might treat yourself immediately after each meal, snack, or drink that fits your eating goals:

➢ Designate a specific reward that you will give yourself at the end of each meal, snack or drink that meets your goal. Remember, a treat can be as easy as telling yourself, "great job on this healthy meal!" Or, "I get a trophy for this one!" Reward your "good" behavior by acknowledging that you accomplished something important. By rewarding healthy eating behavior each time it occurs, you are beginning to pair good feelings with healthy food. Repeated pairings like this strengthen neural connections in your brain, and with time, increase the likelihood that you will continue the healthy eating behavior. Isn't that amazing? Celebrating in your mind is a simple treat, available every time, and extremely powerful in helping you change your behavior.

➢ Alternatively, you can give yourself a star or a point following each healthy meal, snack, or drink. Track these treats on your monitoring chart and decide how many stars or points you need to get a special bonus reward such as a movie night, manicure, or massage. The idea is to treat yourself each time you do the behavior you set out to do. Immediate stars or points need to be recognized as the treat. (You can't get a massage after every healthy meal!) Accumulated points can be "cashed in" for a larger, tangible reward as long as you treat yourself every time along the way.

You now have a game plan for sticking with any eating plan. You have everything you need to succeed. It's time to look forward and envision yourself as a healthier and happier person. Applying this game plan means you have begun to take control of your health destiny.

8

My Exercise Game Plan

The What—Important Information about Your Exercise Program

We have said many times that there is no magic pill, but when it comes to being healthy, physical activity along with a healthy diet is the closest we can get. Let's review some facts from Physical Activity: The Magic Pill, a booklet published by The President's Council on Fitness and Sports and the current recommendations from the American College of Sports Medicine (ACSM):

➢ Moderate physical activity helps lower cholesterol, blood sugar, and blood pressure.

➢ Exercise strengthens muscles and improves flexibility and range of motion, thereby protecting the joints against osteoporosis. It also relieves the symptoms of arthritis.

➢ Physical exercise reduces your risk of cardiovascular disease, stroke, and certain kinds of cancer. It also helps reduce the symptoms of anxiety and depression.

➢ Physical exercise is important for weight management and essential for maintaining weight loss.

➢ Physical activity recommendations are moderate intensity aerobic exercise at least 5 days per week for a total of 150 minutes (30 minutes 5 days/week) to realize *health effects*.

We often hear about "moderate" levels of activity, but it can be difficult to figure out exactly what this means. Here are some examples of light, moderate, and heavy physical activity:

Sedentary

Watching television
Reading
Eating
Typing on the computer
Talking on the phone
Standing in line
Riding in a car
General office work

Light

Slow walking
Cooking food
Washing dishes
Putting away groceries
Child care
Croquet
Mild stretching
Billiards

Moderate

Brisk walking
Weight lifting
Tai chi
Golf
Cleaning house
Gardening
Playing softball

Vigorous

Walking up stairs
Jogging/running
Bicycling (faster than12 mph)
Swimming
Cross-country skiing
Singles tennis
Jumping rope
Playing basketball

ACTION TIP

Get the Ball Rolling

We all know we need to exercise regularly, but it can be so hard to get started.

➤ You need a specific goal—saying you're going to exercise is not specific enough.
➤ Walking for 30 minutes on Monday, Wednesday, and Friday from 5:00 to 5:30 PM is specific. The more specific the goal, the more likely you are to succeed.
➤ Be realistic. Don't set goals that are too big and therefore unattainable. Pick reasonable goals that you can reach. Start small, be successful, and gradually build, and you'll be on your way in developing a healthy exercise habit.

The Want—Are You Motivated to Exercise?

It's time to focus on exercise and be honest about your desire to change. Do you to want to make changes in your exercise regimen in order to improve your health? Are you motivated to change your exercise level—whether this means starting to exercise or increasing the amount of exercise you do? How important is it to you to exercise? If your answer is "no," or "it's not important," you probably won't be able to make lasting changes in your exercise behaviors, and this isn't a good time to begin a new program. You may be able to find your internal motivation to be healthier by answering the questions in Chapter 3. Review what we said about motivation.

If your answer to this question is "yes" and that exercise is important to you—great! You have some degree of motivation to change your behavior and keep it going over the long term. Let's examine more closely the degree to which you're motivated to change your exercise levels.

Rate your level of motivation on this scale:

1	2	3	4	5	6	7	8	9	10

Not motivated   Completely motivated

If your degree of motivation is 3 or less, go back to Chapter 3 and use the motivation-boosting strategies. Exercise and physical activity need to be important to you. You need to be able to identify the benefits of it and clarify the reasons that it would make a difference for you and your health.

If you rated your motivation as 4 or higher, you're ready to get started. Remember, you don't have to be a "10"—completely motivated. Even if you rate yourself at midpoint on the scale, you have enough motivation to start your new exercise program. We've said it earlier; motivation typically comes and goes over time depending on the behavior, the person, and the situation. Whenever you feel your motivation level getting low, go back and use the boosters in Chapter 3.

The How—SMART Skills for Making Exercise Happen

You've got The What and The Want, but how do you make exercise a reality? Here are some specific examples of SMART skills that focus on exercise. Read through them to learn about how to start your new exercise routine.

Set a Goal. There are endless possibilities when it comes to physical activity. As you might imagine, we couldn't even begin to think of all the possible exercise goals. However, most people seem to share some common objectives. We also find that the changes people want to make follow some general themes, such as "I want to do aerobic exercise every day," "I want to get stronger," or "I want to improve the way my body looks."

These are wonderful ideas, but they are far too general. As we have noted elsewhere, setting a goal means identifying a specific behavior that can be changed. Your goal needs to be observable and measurable. The more specific, observable, and measurable the goal, the more likely you are to succeed. Your goal also needs to be one that you feel confident that you can achieve. How could you make the goal "I want to do aerobic exercise every day" specific, observable, and measurable? Write your answers below.

General goal: "I want to do aerobic exercise every day."

Make it specific: _____

_____

How could you observe it? _____

_____.

How could you measure it? _____

_____.

One specific exercise might be to walk on a treadmill for 30 minutes every day of the workweek, with weekends off. Aerobic exercise is not a specific behavior, but walking on a treadmill can be observed, and you can time how long you walk during each exercise session. Whether you walk on a treadmill or at a track, in the park or at the mall, walking is one of the easiest exercises you can do, but be sure to keep track of your time using a watch or stopwatch.

Should you start at 30 minutes right off the bat? Probably not, if you haven't been walking at all. Remember, your goal is to reach a level where you are walking 5 days a week for 30 minutes at a time. If you are just getting started, the most important thing you can do is to make sure you succeed. This is the concept of pacing, which we talked about earlier. Let's take another look at pacing.

If you think you can walk for 30 minutes, but aren't sure, what might happen? You will probably make it through the first day without much difficulty. What happens if you wake up the next morning and are sore and worn out? Your chances of walking again the second day go way down. You might skip the next walking session, and then you are off to a poor start toward your exercise goal.

In order to guarantee that each exercise session is a success, take the amount of exercise you know you can do and cut it in half for the first week. If you know you can do 30 minutes, walk for no more and no less than 15 minutes for the first week of your new target behavior. Each week, add 5 more minutes to your walking, no more and no less.

Your exercise time will look like this:

Week 1   15 minutes
Week 2   20 minutes
Week 3   25 minutes
Week 4   30 minutes

Once you have reached the 30-minute goal, you can add more time or walk more quickly. The most important concept here is that, you need to develop the habit of exercise before you will be able to improve your physical conditioning.

Monitor Your Progress. Monitoring your exercise takes some effort, but we know that monitoring behavior changes behavior. You have a number of options for keeping track. You can take your monitoring chart with you when you walk at a gym, and simply mark off the time you started walking and the time you finished. You can do the same thing with a phone app. You could also wait and fill in the monitoring chart at home after you have completed your walk. As you gradually increase your level of activity, be sure to notice these improvements. If you find it helpful, you can get "fancy" by graphing your progress over the weeks and months. Finally, be sure to post the chart in a visible place to remind you of your goal and your weekly progress.

Arrange Your World for Success. This SMART skill will help you create an environment that will support your exercise goals. The idea is to make it as easy as possible to do the behavior you've targeted. When you don't arrange your world, all kinds of things get in your way: getting up late, forgetting where you put your workout clothes, not having enough time to exercise and still get to your job on time, bad weather, or an unexpected appointment. The obstacles seem to jump out at you from every direction. By arranging your world and planning ahead, you can head off these problems before they stop you from exercising. Here are a few suggestions that will help you set up your surroundings to make it easy to do the right thing:

> ➢ Select a time that fits into your schedule that you can exercise on the days you set.
> ➢ Put the time in your calendar—make an appointment with yourself for exercising.
> ➢ Have your walking shoes and anything else that you need for exercising ready to go. When your time comes, you don't want to be scrambling to get things together.
> ➢ If you exercise first thing in the morning, set your alarm clock to get out of bed. It is a simple way to arrange your world, and can make all the difference.
> ➢ If you need support from others, be sure you have it in place.

Recruit a Support Team. Working out with a partner makes exercise fun and adds external accountability, so:

> ➢ Tell family, friends, and co-workers that you are starting an exercise program and ask if they will join you.
> ➢ Look for people at the park or gym who are exercising by themselves at the same time as you. They might be perfect partners. When you find exercise partners, make sure they are as committed to exercising as you are.
> ➢ Tell your spouse or significant other you need help in sticking with it (for example, giving you time to exercise, watching the children, joining you in the workout).
> ➢ Let your supporters know exactly how they can help you be successful.

Treat Yourself. Let's face it: Many people who start an exercise program do it because they need to improve their health, rather than because they see it as fun. It will take a while, but once you develop the exercise habit, you will enjoy it, look forward to it, and even crave it. It may not be so rewarding when you first start, so it is critical that you give yourself treats as a reward to keep going.

Here are a few suggestions for treats:

➤ After every exercise session, tell yourself "congratulations, I did it!" or give yourself a high five for meeting your goal. This is an immediate, powerful treat, which works.

➤ Treat yourself to new workout shoes, apparel, or equipment, after you have met your exercise goals for a few weeks. Use the point system to treat yourself each time you exercise and use your accumulated points for something tangible.

➤ Treat yourself to a few minutes in the sauna, steam room, or Jacuzzi after an exercise session. Or decide in advance that your treat will be an uninterrupted shower or bath at home.

➤ Put gold stars on your monitoring chart after each workout. As we've said before, this sounds silly, but it works.

The particular treat you choose is not as important as making sure you schedule it for after you finish exercising. Treats help you pair good feelings with exercise and building rewards into your routine will help your exercise program become a permanent habit. Once it has become a habit, you can treat yourself intermittently. We still give ourselves a "high five" every time after an exercise session because it is an easy treat and it always feels good.

Exercise is a lifelong activity. Lifelong, however, doesn't mean every single day for the rest of your life. This game plan will provide you the specifics you need to get your exercise program up and running, and stick with it. If you miss a workout, no problem. Just focus on exercising more days than not as your long-term, lifestyle goal.

ACTION TIP

Parents: Fit Exercise into Your Schedule

Parents are some of the busiest people in the world, and their hectic schedules often leave little time for exercise. Here are four tips to help you fit exercise into your day:

➢ Examine your schedule hour by hour. You'll be surprised by how many gaps of 15–20 minutes you actually have to squeeze in some physical activity.

➢ Do double duty. Walk around the soccer field while the kids are practicing, or walk or jog in the neighborhood where their piano lessons are taught.

➢ You probably have a friend or neighbor who is as busy as you are. Set up a "kid swap," where you each agree to watch each other's kids while the other exercises.

➢ Finally, ask your spouse or significant other to take care of the kids while you exercise.

➢ These strategies may not get you into the gym every day, but they will help you become more active.

9

My Sleep Game Plan

The What—Important Information about Sleep

We all know what it feels like to not get a good night's sleep. Poor sleep is a nightly reality for many people. A 2014 poll by the National Sleep Foundation found that up to 45 percent of adult Americans reported sleep problems that affected their daily lives in at least one of the past seven days. The National Highway Traffic Safety Administration estimates that each year up to 100,000 police-reported accidents involve drowsiness.

Research clearly suggests that poor-quality sleep can put you at greater risk for diminished work productivity, anxiety and depression, and motor vehicle accidents, as well as increased risk for colon and breast cancer, heart disease, and diabetes (Institute of Medicine 2006). This means that improving your quality of sleep is a reasonable and important lifestyle goal.

The Want—Are You Motivated to Change Your Sleep Habits?

Most people who suffer from the effects of poor sleep really do want better quality sleep. However, getting a good night's sleep requires you to change some of your current habits. You will have to do things differently, and so we are back to this important question: Are you motivated to change your routines in a way that will result in better sleep? Or, "what concerns do you have about your current sleep patterns?" If your answer is "no," or that you aren't concerned, this is probably not a good time for you to try to do something to improve your sleep habits. The principles and the SMART skills will still be here when you find yourself a little more motivated to change. You can always go back to Chapter 3 to decide whether you really want to change.

If your answer to this question is "yes"—great! You have The Want to make changes in your sleep habits in order to get better quality sleep.

Let's examine more closely the degree to which you're motivated to change your sleep-related routines. Rate your level of motivation on the scale below.

1	2	3	4	5	6	7	8	9	10

Not motivated   Completely motivated

If your degree of motivation is 3 or less, go back to Chapter 3 and use the motivation-boosting strategies. It's important to consider the benefits of better sleep and find your own reasons why improved sleep is important. If you rated your motivation as 4 or greater, you're ready to get started. As we've said before, you don't have to be a "10"—completely motivated. If you rate yourself at midpoint on the scale, you have enough motivation to start changing your sleep habits. Whenever you feel your motivation waning, go back and complete the motivational exercises in Chapter 3 for a boost.

The How—SMART Skills for Improving Your Sleep

You know that sleep is important, and you want to improve the quality of your sleep by changing your sleep-related routines. Now that you've got The What and The Want, it's time to make The How a reality. The following specific examples of SMART skills focus on sleep. Read them to learn about how to start your new sleep routine.

Set a Goal. You say you want better sleep. Seems straightforward enough, doesn't it? Let's stop for a minute and be more specific. What do you really want? Do you want to sleep more hours? Do you want to go to bed earlier? Get up earlier? Go to bed and stay asleep all night? There are many possible goals. To make sure you reach your true sleep goal, you must be specific about what you want. Then you need to be specific about what behaviors you need to change in order to reach that goal. Everything must be measurable and observable. "Better sleep" is not measurable or observable. Goals such as sleeping through the night without waking up, sleeping for 8 hours, 5 nights a week, and going to bed at 9:30 P.M. are all specific, observable, and measurable actions. However, they are still a bit too general. How do you make the goal "sleep for 8 hours" as specific as possible? Give it a try below.

General goal: "I want to sleep for 8 hours."

Make it specific: _____

_____.

How could you observe it? _____

_____.

How could you measure it? _____

_____.

Here's what we came up with as possible goals you could use:

➢ Get ready for bed at 8:00 P.M.
➢ Wind down with a cup of decaffeinated tea or read a book.
➢ Go into the bedroom at approximately 9:15 P.M.
➢ Set the alarm for 5:45 A.M.
➢ Allow 30 minutes to fall asleep.

These times and sleep routines may not fit exactly with your preferences, but the idea is to develop a detailed plan for what is necessary for you to reach your goal of sleeping for 8 hours.

Monitor Your Progress. Monitoring your sleep progress really translates into creating a sleep log, or diary. Whether it's a notebook, a calendar, or a phone app, try to monitor the following categories:

> ➢ The time you went to bed.
> ➢ How sleepy you felt when you went to bed—use a 0–10 scale, with 0 being "not sleepy at all" and 10 being "extremely sleepy."
> ➢ In the morning, note the time you woke up (not what time you got out of bed).
> ➢ How refreshed/rested you felt—use the same 0–10 scale, with 0 being "not rested at all" and 10 being "extremely rested."
> ➢ How many times you remember waking up during the night and approximately how long you were awake.

Using these categories, your sleep log for one night might look something like this:

Sleep Monitoring Chart for Sunday/Monday

My goal is 8 hours of sleep each night.

Wake Time Sunday_____

How refreshed (0–10) _____

Number of times woke up Sunday night _____

Bedtime Monday night _____

How Sleepy (0–10) _____

Continue to monitor your sleep progress, and you should see improvement within a week or so.

Arrange Your World for Success. Sleep is a behavior, and although it can be influenced by many medical conditions, the actions you take prior to sleeping will have a great impact on how well you sleep.

Here are some basic guidelines to arrange your surroundings for better sleep:

➤ Go to bed and get up at a similar time every day. This may be more challenging on the weekends, but by using an alarm clock you can make sure your sleep cycle has a regular rhythm, which will help improve your sleep.

➤ Use your bed for only for sleeping. Don't use it for watching television, paying bills, or working. That way, when you go to bed, your body will know it's time to sleep.

➤ Reduce any noise in your room. If you can't reduce the noise, consider getting a "white noise" machine or foam ear plugs.

➤ Make sure your bed and bedroom are quiet and comfortable, and slightly cool. A hot room can disrupt sleep. A cool room and enough blankets to keep warm if needed are best.

➤ Set up a sleep routine you can follow every night. These are simply actions that you engage in to help you unwind. It's important to give your body cues that it's time to slow down and sleep. Try listening to relaxing music, read something soothing for 15 minutes, or practice meditation or prayer. Anything that calms you down and makes you drowsy is good. Be sure to practice the routine every night, regardless of how sleepy you are.

➤ Don't drink caffeine or alcohol, smoke, or exercise 4–6 hours before bedtime, because it can interfere with the quality of sleep.

➤ Don't take naps. You want to be tired at bedtime. If you can't make it through the day without a nap, sleep less than 1 hour and take your nap before 3 P.M.

➤ Finally, if you can't fall asleep, don't stay in your bed for more than 20 minutes. Instead, get up, go into a dimly lit room and do something restful, such as listen to quiet music. Get back into bed when you feel sleepy.

Recruit a Support Team. Recruiting a support team is critical if you sleep with another person, because your efforts to improve your sleep may significantly change your current sleep habits, and that, in turn, can affect the sleep of a spouse or significant other. Communication with your sleep partner is essential.

Before you make changes, talk to the person you live with. Let your partner know what your goal is, why you would want to make changes to your current routines, and why her help is important to your success. Be open to compromise. A 9:15 P.M. bedtime may be great for you, but it may not be for your sleep partner. Discuss how you can make it work for both of you. It may take your going to bed first and your significant other watching television in another room instead of the bedroom. Remember, if you want help and support, you need to be clear about what you want the other person to do, and be willing to compromise.

Treat Yourself. Getting a good night's sleep is one of those behaviors that is rewarding once it starts to happen. As we have all experienced, there is nothing better than feeling completely refreshed when you wake up. As you begin to develop better sleep habits and your sleep improves, you will feel rejuvenated and rewarded. However, there is benefit to a reward in the form of gold stars on your sleep log, telling yourself, "great job" when you are on schedule, or even a special treat at the end of the week if you do what you set out to do.

The better you sleep, the better you will feel. For most people, changing some of their night time routines is all that is needed. It may take some time, so give it a few weeks. Remember, sleep problems may be the sign of a more serious medical problem. Consult your doctor if changes in your routines don't seem to be helping.

10

My Medication Game Plan

The What—Important Information about Taking Medication

Did you know that 32 million Americans take three or more medications daily? It's estimated that 75 percent of them take their medication improperly (National Council on Patient Information and Education, 2014). Whether it's taking too much, not enough, not completing a prescription, or not refilling a prescription, medication nonadherence has significant effects on health. Tens of thousands of deaths, numerous hospitalizations, and delayed recovery from illnesses occur each year because people don't take their medications properly (Osterberg & Blaschke, 2005).

Here are some statistics from the National Pharmaceutical Council, the American Hospital Association, and the American Heart Association:

> ➤ Medication nonadherence results in more than 125,000 deaths a year—twice as many people as are killed in motor vehicle accidents.

➢ People who regularly miss medication doses visit the doctor three times as much as those who take their medication as prescribed.

➢ Ten percent of all hospital admissions are the result of not taking prescription medications as prescribed.

➢ The average hospital stay due to medication nonadherence is 4.2 days.

➢ Twenty-three percent of all nursing home admissions are due to failure to take medications correctly.

Some of the most common behavioral errors people make when it comes to taking medication include:

➢ Forgetting to take medication.
➢ Stopping before a medication prescription is finished.
➢ Taking the wrong dose.
➢ Taking extra doses when a dose is missed.
➢ Taking medication with the wrong food or drink.
➢ Taking medication with other prescriptions or over-the-counter drugs, which can produce side effects.
➢ Not filling or refilling a prescription.

Taking medications as prescribed can be challenging, especially if you need to take them for a long period of time. Taking medication daily is required for many conditions, including heart disease, high blood pressure, high cholesterol, some types of asthma, and HIV-AIDS. Taking medication on a regular basis is a behavior that can be developed into a habit, similar to changing your eating or exercise habits.

The Want—Am I Committed to Taking My Medication?

Most people say they are motivated to take a prescribed medication if it makes them feel better, improves their health, prevents an illness, or prolongs their lives. Are you motivated? Are you willing to make changes in your habits to make sure you will take your medication properly? Are you willing to endure the possible side effects of the medication, manage the costs associated with taking it, and deal with possible disruptions in your life that taking the medication may cause?

If your answer to this question is "yes"—great! You understand that some degree of motivation is necessary to change behavior and to keep it going over the long term, and you have The Want to make changes in your routines in order to be successful. If your answer to this question is "no," that you don't really see the benefits from taking medications, you're not likely to succeed in changing your behavior in order to take your medication properly. It's time to figure out why taking your medication might be important to you. Below is one of the exercises from Chapter 3 that may help you tap into your intrinsic motivation to be healthier and decide whether taking medication as prescribed would be beneficial to you. Even if you completed this exercise earlier, try it again and focus specifically on the issue of taking medication.

Ask yourself these questions and write down the answers:

What is the relationship between taking your prescribed medications and your long-term health? _____
_____.

What behaviors are you doing to ensure that you take your medications as recommended?
_____
_____.

What would be better for your health if you were able to make improvements in your medication routine? _____
_____.

What other benefits would you expect?_____
_____.

By taking the time to answer these questions, most people will be reminded of why they wanted to make changes in the first place. Simple as it seems, these questions can really boost your level of motivation and remind you about what is important to you. So, if you ever find your motivation slipping, return to Chapter 3 and repeat this exercise.

Now, let's examine more closely the degree to which you're motivated to stick with your medication regimen. Rate your level of motivation on the scale below.

1   2   3   4   5   6   7   8   9   10

Not motivated   Completely motivated

If your degree of motivation is 3 or less, go back to Chapter 3 and use the additional motivation-boosting strategies, including the one just given above. It's important to find your internal motivation and your own reasons for why you want to take your medication as recommended.

If you rated your motivation as 4 or greater, you're ready to get started. Remember, you don't have to be a "10"—completely motivated. If you rate yourself at mid-point on the scale, you still have enough motivation to start changing your medication habits. As we talked about earlier, you can expect your motivation to come and go over time. Whenever you feel your motivation level decreasing, go back and use the booster exercises and remind yourself about what you really want.

The How—SMART Skills for Taking Your Medication Consistently

Below are specific examples of SMART skills that focus on taking medication. Read through them to learn about how to stay on track with your medication regimen.

Set a Goal. Much like sleep, setting a goal for medication seems quite straightforward. "I want to take my medication as prescribed" is a reasonable goal. However, as with all the behaviors we have already discussed, "taking my medication as prescribed" is neither observable nor measurable. At this point you may be thinking: "Of course, I can take medication properly." Right? Not really. Taking medication as it is prescribed involves developing a series of specific behaviors that are observable and measurable.

Try this exercise. How could you make the goal, "I want to take my medication as prescribed" specific, observable, and measurable? Write your answers below.

General goal: "I want to take my medication as my doctor prescribed it."

Make it specific: _____
_____.

How could you observe it? _____
_____.

How could you measure it? _____
_____.

While every medication regimen will differ, here are the specific behaviors we came up with that could define taking medication as prescribed:

> Taking the right amount (number of pills).
> Taking it at the right times (number of times a day).
> Taking it with or without the right foods (empty stomach, with a meal, with or without dairy products).
> Taking it with or without other medications.
> Taking it for the right amount of time (10 days vs. ongoing).

Each of these is observable, and together they will result in the goal of taking the medication properly. Now look back at your specific goal. Did you include all the necessary behaviors? If so, it's time to move on to the next SMART skill. If not, make it more specific and then move on.

Monitor Your Progress. There are several ways to create a medication diary, or log, to monitor your progress. A wall calendar or The Chart will work just fine. Each day, simply write down the name of the medication, the time you took it, and the amount you took. Put the calendar or chart somewhere near the medication, such as in the bathroom. The US Department of Health and Human Services, Food and Drug Administration offers a free medication

JOSHUA KLAPOW, SHERI PRUITT

monitoring chart, which can be downloaded at: https://www.fda.gov/downloads/AboutFDA/ReportsManualsForms/Forms/UCM095018.pdf

Arrange Your World for Success. There are so many opportunities to not take medication—from forgetting, to running out, to not having it with you at the proper time. By arranging your world for success, you can set up your environment to make it easy to do the right thing. Here are some strategies that can help you arrange your environment to increase the chances of taking your medication at the right time and in the right amount:

- ➢ Take medication with daily activities, such as eating breakfast or brushing your teeth.
- ➢ Use a pillbox with separate compartments for each day. They are inexpensive and can be purchased at most pharmacies. Place it on a counter where you can see it.
- ➢ Set an alarm on your phone.
- ➢ Plan ahead for travel by filling a separate pill box.

Recruit a Support Team. Taking your medication safely and consistently will help keep you healthy. This has direct benefits to your spouse, partner, family, friends, co-workers, employer, community, and even your pets. Getting help from the people around you is well justified. One of the simplest actions you can take is to let everyone you are comfortable with or have a close relationship with know that you need to take your medication regularly. Ask them to remind you or to check with you to be sure you took it. People who care about you will be happy to support and encourage you.

In addition to friends and family, you can create what we call a medication support team. Your team could include your doctor or nurse practitioner, a care manager if you are participating in a disease management program, and your pharmacist. Although they may not remind you to take your medication, they can play a critical role in helping you take it safely. Make sure all the members of your health care team know what medicines you are taking (both prescription and over-the-counter), and always report side effects to them. Always check with your doctor before stopping or changing a medication.

Your pharmacy can also play a helpful role. Try to see the same pharmacist each time you fill or refill a prescription. You can ask her about taking over-the-counter medications with your prescriptions, and she can help clarify possible interactions between medications and between certain kinds of food and medications. With the help of your family, friends, and medication support team, you will be more successful in making changes in your habits and routines needed to stick with your medication regimen.

ACTION TIP

The Basics of Managing a Chronic Illness

From diabetes to heart disease to asthma, chronic conditions affect over half of all American adults. That's 117 million people. When you are trying to juggle medications, doctor's visits, and everything else that is involved in managing a chronic disease, changing your diet and exercising can easily become overwhelming. Despite this, some simple actions that will help you manage any chronic condition include:

➤ Learn what behaviors are important in managing your chronic illness. Consider medications, diet, exercise, tracking of symptoms, and anything else your health care provider recommends.
➤ Stay healthy. Eating well, exercising regularly, and getting enough sleep will increase your ability to cope with and manage your condition.
➤ Stress can make your condition worse and make you less likely to do the healthy behaviors you need to do, so take time to relax and manage stress.
➤ Ask your family, friends, and health care providers to support you.
➤ Follow your doctor's instructions, especially about how to take the medications for your illness.

Treat Yourself. Why should you treat yourself for taking your medication properly? Some medications will make you feel better, and when you feel better, you are being rewarded or "treated." Feeling good after taking a medication makes it easier for this behavior to be repeated -- to take the medication on a regular basis. An aspirin that makes a headache go away or an antacid that soothes your stomach have built-in rewards in that they relieve your symptoms.

However, the medications used to treat conditions such as high cholesterol, high blood pressure, and depression are not likely to make you feel better immediately. Because of this, taking them doesn't give you any noticeable reward. Some medications, such as certain antiviral agents for HIV-AIDS and chemotherapy for cancer, don't make you feel better immediately, and the side effects can make you feel worse. However, most people feel that taking these medications is valuable because they promote health in the long run. The challenge in taking medication for a long period of time is that it's easy to forget until it becomes a habit. This is where having a reward or treat schedule to get the behavior going is essential.

If you have to take medication daily for an indefinite period of time, you need to make sure you are rewarded for doing it. Much as with exercise or diet, simply pick a treat that you will give yourself after taking your medication every time.

The trick is to pick something that can be immediate and makes you feel good about what you've done. Here are a few suggestions:

> Treat yourself by telling yourself, "great job!" Saying something, even inside your head, can be a very powerful reward.

> Treat yourself with a point on your monitoring chart. Get points for each time you take your medications as prescribed and at the end of the week, go out or rent a special movie if you met your medication goal.

> Put gold stars on your monitoring chart each time after successfully taking your medication. Look at all your stars and feel good about your progress.

While it seems simple enough, many people fail to develop good habits for taking medication. When you have turned the act of taking your medication into a habit, you won't have to worry about forgetting to take it and you will improve your health. In some cases, you might even save your life.

PART 3

Get Help When You Need It

Even with the best of intentions and the most carefully laid plans, we all get stuck from time to time when we're trying to change. While the circumstances and specific behaviors may differ from person to person, there seems to be a set of sticking points that most people run into. This section is designed to help you get past them.

You may not need this kind of help right now, and if you don't—good for you. However, if you find yourself struggling at any point to make the changes you need to or want to make, read the stories in this section. You'll see how we work with people struggling with the most common sticking points. This is how we help them break through the major blocks and move closer toward their goals.

11

When Life Gets Tough: Coaching Sessions with Drs. Klapow and Pruitt

You have everything you need to make changes in any health behavior. By now, you can say "information, motivation, and SMART skills" in your sleep. However, you may be thinking, "Easier said than done," and, in a way, you're right. Knowing what to change, wanting to change, and having the SMART skills will help you be successful in making behavioral changes, but you will probably face challenges along the way. Almost everyone does.

Sometimes it can be helpful to see how other people have overcome their problems. The stories below are from some of our clients who wanted to make changes in their daily health habits, but were having difficulty. Read about their struggles, their successes, and how our coaching tips helped them to get over some of these hurdles. Test yourself, too. Fill in the spaces provided with your own advice about how to make successful behavioral changes.

> Marie: "I'm completely motivated to get back to my exercise routine after having a baby, but this is not working. Before having a child, I was very active and I felt good. Why am I stuck? Why can't I get back on track?"

Marie is a married, 27-year-old woman who has recently undergone two major life events: She graduated with a degree in veterinary medicine and had her first child. While pregnant, Marie felt free from following any serious constraints about eating, and she enjoyed many foods she had previously banished from her diet. She also hit "pause" on her exercise routine. The extra weight and fatigue near the end of her pregnancy made it difficult to be active.

Throughout her life, Marie had struggled with consistent exercise, but just before her pregnancy, she found her rhythm. She had been training for a 5K race in San Diego with her girlfriends. For the first time, the trip and the goal of the fun run helped Marie stick to an exercise plan. She was making good progress with jogging 3 days a week. The later stages of the pregnancy put this on hold.

Marie gained about 10 pounds while pregnant, but closely watched her diet and her scale following the birth of her baby. During the first 4 weeks she was thrilled to see that she was losing weight, but she became disappointed as time passed, because she wasn't having success with getting back to her exercise regimen. Her friends were planning to enter another fun run in the next few months and she didn't want to miss out. She just couldn't get back on track.

Marie recalled going through phases during which she would exercise consistently for a few weeks, stop for a while, and then start again, but she felt she wasn't making much progress and wouldn't be able to keep up with her friends. Moreover, Marie wanted to incorporate exercise into her life permanently so she could feel good about her weight and be as healthy as possible. Having a baby made Marie take a lot of things more seriously. She was motivated to make some changes for her own health, and she also wanted to be healthy for her new child.

Marie read this book, completed the interactive exercises, and was ready to get started. She set a short-term goal of walking briskly on her treadmill 3 days a week (Monday, Wednesday, and Friday) for 30 minutes from 6:30 to 7:00 A.M.

She met this goal the first week, but only walked 1 day each during the second and third weeks. By the fourth week she had completely stopped. We met with Marie to find out what had gone wrong. Here's what she said:

"I was eager to get going on my exercise program. I was really motivated to get back to where I was before my pregnancy and dedicate myself to getting and staying healthy. I read your book and followed your advice. I set a goal that was specific and not too difficult. I cleared the stack of boxes from my treadmill and arranged my environment just as you suggested. I even had my daily reward built in—I was going to treat myself by listening to one of my favorite podcasts during my walk. I did everything just as you said. The first week went just great. Then the second week, my son was up for 2 nights in a row, and I was simply too tired to do any exercise. By the third week, each morning just seemed to slip by, and although I did walk on one day, the rest of the week was crazy. By the fourth week, I thought about using the tread-mill every day, but for whatever reason, I just didn't do it. This is so frustrating. I really want to get in shape to do the next fun run with my girlfriends. I couldn't be more motivated. Why is it so easy to forget or to do just about anything else other than walk on that darned treadmill?"

We asked Marie to think about the three key questions: Do you know what to do? Do you want to do it? Do you know how to change your behavior? She knew she had to walk on the treadmill to get in shape; she clearly wanted to do it, but somehow it just wasn't happening. Marie said, "Yes, I know what to do; yes, I want to do it; and yes, I now know how to change my routine. Why am I still having a problem?"

Marie's use of the SMART skills seemed worthy of a closer look. Marie had set a specific and achievable goal, arranged her environment for success, and had decided on an easy way to treat herself for meeting her daily walking goal. That left two SMART skills that Marie didn't mention: monitoring progress and recruiting a support team.

We asked Marie about her support team. She was clear about her husband's support. "My husband is 100 percent behind me on this. He agreed to watch our son and has been encouraging." It sounded like Marie had a reasonably good support team in her husband, but what about monitoring? She said that she photocopied The Chart out of the book, but she admitted she didn't use it because it didn't seem necessary just to track 30 minutes of walking in her own home.

If you were coaching Marie about what to do to increase her chances of being successful with using her treadmill, what tips would you give her?

_____

_____

_____

_____

Did you suggest that Marie monitor her progress? This SMART skill seems to be the one she had overlooked. The tendency to discount the power of monitoring is something we see all the time. Keeping a close watch on behavior is especially important for counting calories, reducing the number of cigarettes you smoke, or keeping track of a complicated workout routine. But when the behavior is something as simple as walking once a day, keeping track of it on paper seems a bit unnecessary because it's so easy to remember if you did it or not.

However, this is where many people go wrong. Keeping track of your actions isn't only about remembering what you did. In fact, the power in monitoring what you do is that it increases the likelihood of your changing – monitoring behavior changes behavior. Marie had a specific and measurable goal. She had arranged her world and had support and a reward schedule, but she had no visual cue or reminder to walk on her treadmill each morning. There was nothing to demonstrate the progress she was making in meeting her goal or help her be accountable.

Marie needed to think about changing her routine as a game of probabilities. She should be doing everything possible to increase her chances of doing the behavior (in this situation, walking on the treadmill) and decrease the chances that she won't. What happened to Marie is a demonstration of the need for a set of skills—not just one or two— in order to maximize the chances of being successful in making lasting behavioral changes. The SMART skills seem so simple and straightforward that people often underestimate the impact each one can have on behavior.

Marie found it difficult to believe that not monitoring her progress was the reason she was struggling with her walking program. She needed to be reminded of the power of this SMART skill. Her monitoring chart should be placed in a highly visible location. When she sees it, Marie will be forced to make a conscious decision between walking on the treadmill or not. Without a reminder or visual cue in your environment, it's easy for old habits, routines, and thoughts to take over. If Marie has a monitoring chart on the refrigerator and notices it every time she passes by, she will be much more likely to get on the treadmill. Monitoring her walking will help keep her accountable. She will see exactly how she's doing--in black and white. After Marie tracks her progress for a week or two, and recognizes how much she's accomplished, it will be difficult to stop moving toward her goal.

Marie is one of the most motivated people we've met. She really wanted to exercise and improve her health. Her story is a great example of the need for more than willpower, desire, or strong motivation to change behavior. It's easy to be motivated for a week or so, but motivation alone won't pull you through. It simply isn't enough to keep new behaviors going. All the SMART skills have to be included in your plan to ensure the best chance of success. Good health doesn't happen just because you really want it, but there isn't any magic involved, either.

Susan is experiencing "the Drift."
"I've tried this before and it doesn't work," she said. "There has to be a better way."

It seems to happen every year. On New Year's Eve, Susan sets the goal of getting in shape for the annual beach vacation she takes with her husband each summer. She knows the SMART skills and for a while, follows them closely, but by March, Susan is slipping back into her old patterns.

Susan is 56 years old. She is generally healthy, but over the past 10 years she has become less active, has eaten more than she needs, and has gained about 20 pounds. She knows she should watch her diet more closely and exercise regularly, and every January she starts off with a bang. In fact, for the past 5 years, Susan has lost about 10 pounds every year between January and April by following a strict eating and exercise plan. She strives for perfection, and rarely has a day in which she doesn't meet her eating and activity goals. Susan says her problem is that no matter how motivated she seems to be in January, her motivation fades by March, and she just can't seem to hold on to lifestyle changes into the summer months. Here's what Susan said when we met with her:

_____
_____
_____
_____

"I'm at my wit's end. This happens every year. I start the year really motivated and make good progress, but everything seems to fade away by spring. I don't understand how I can lose weight by exercising and eating right, and then by spring, bingo, I'm back to square one and the weight returns. I've tried this behavioral stuff so many times before. It just doesn't work."

Susan is experiencing a pattern that happens to a lot of people. They start out strong, apply all of the SMART skills, and have good success for a short period of time. Then, something happens and they begin to lose their motivation. A number of our clients tell us they feel just as Susan does—that they're "back to square one." Susan needed to hear the good news: Her problem can be identified and resolved.

Although it may seem like "bingo" and "back to square one" to Susan, let's examine this a bit more closely. Susan agreed that it took several weeks to lose those 10 pounds and get in the routine of regular exercise. Also, she agreed that it was physically impossible to gain the 10 pounds she had lost in a day. Even if Susan were to stop the eating and exercising changes she was making, it would be at least a few weeks until she gained back all of the weight she had lost. Thus, she has time to heed a warning.

If you were Susan's behavioral change coach, what would you suggest to help her sustain the gains she had made over the first 3 months? What seems to be happening to her?

_____

_____

_____

_____

Maybe Susan's problem isn't that the SMART skills "just don't work." Maybe she needs to review Chapter 5, where we discussed behavioral drift. Recall that "drift" describes slipping back into old, more familiar patterns of behavior. In Susan's case, after about 3 months of making behavioral changes, she was slipping back into her old ways of eating too much and exercising too little.

Susan considered the possibility that she might be experiencing behavioral drift. She also entertained the idea that the SMART skills might be effective if she kept doing them. Although Susan somewhat agreed with what we were saying, she clearly wasn't convinced. We forged ahead.

The good news for Susan was that her problem was easy to solve. She simply needed to catch herself drifting back into her old patterns. If she could use the "three-day rule" (see Chapter 5) to catch herself early, she would be able to get back on track and meet her goal.

Susan wanted to know what was so important about 3 days. We told her this was her "red flag," a signal to stop and find out why she was getting off-track and not meeting her eating and activity goals. We emphasized that the beauty of the three-day rule was that it would allow her to end the backward slide and prevent any significant weight gain (remembering that no one can gain 10 pounds in 3 days). If Susan catches herself in the first three days of getting off-track and corrects her course, she will not regain the weight she's lost. Although she understood the importance of the three-day rule, Susan still was concerned that her enthusiasm for sticking with her new behaviors seemed to fade fairly quickly, and that all seemed to be lost once it faded. For Susan, the solution was to catch problems early by being alert to the onset of behavioral drift and sustaining some level of motivation across time.

What coaching tips would you give Susan about motivation and how to keep it going over time?

_____

_____

_____

_____

For most people, motivation for making behavioral changes tends to wax and wane. Motivation is dynamic over time, and as a result, it requires some ongoing attention. There are several effective strategies that will keep motivation going. One is to remind yourself frequently about your reasons for wanting to eat better or exercise more. Susan should take a minute to consider the following questions:

How do you want to feel 6 months from today? How healthy do you want to be? How do you want to look? Why do you need to be physically fit? How important is this to you? How do you know that you can do it? She might benefit from saying these answers out loud to someone else or writing her answers to these questions on a sheet of paper, so she can review them often to remind herself of the benefits of making lifestyle changes.

More motivational questions for Susan include: What are you doing today to become the person you had in mind when you started making lifestyle changes? What steps are you taking right now to ensure that you become that person? When we asked Susan, she said, "Those questions definitely make me think." "I know how I want to be and I'm not doing the things I need to do to get there."

Susan can also think of motivation as self-perpetuating. By using the SMART skills, she can start a behavioral change cycle in which she initially has a level of motivation to make the desired changes. As she recognizes progress in an area (such as weight loss) her motivation will continue and increase because she likes the experience of success. As Susan continues to use the SMART skills, her confidence will improve, her perceptions of herself will change, she can maintain her motivation, and the positive cycle will perpetuate.

Doing these simple motivational exercises will remind Susan of why she started to make behavioral changes in the first place, and they will give her that little boost of internal motivation she needs to keep going. Motivation can build on itself, too. If Susan will catch problems early, stick with the SMART skills, and think about boosting her motivation and confidence along the way, she can prevent the drift from pulling her back into her old behavior patterns of eating too much and exercising too little. With time and practice, these new eating and exercising behaviors will become more automatic and will take less effort.

Susan's frustration, expressed as "I've tried this before—behavioral stuff just doesn't work," is something we hear a lot. It's not that the SMART skills don't work— but that they work only when you use them. People initially have the motivation to change and they use the SMART skills for a while. At some point, however, motivation declines, nothing is done to replenish it, and a habit has not yet been established. Then, the SMART skills drop out and, eventually, old behavioral patterns reemerge. This experience has a name: "behavioral drift" and drift is something we (and you) know how to address.

All of us are at risk of reverting to old habits when we start making changes in our routines. Initially, we think: "That won't happen to me. I have the motivation to stick with it." In fact, behavioral drift happens to everyone. It is powerful, and if you think about it for a minute, it makes sense. If you've had a habit for 1, 5, or even 10 years, and then try to change it, wouldn't you expect to be pulled back into your long-standing, familiar patterns? These are behaviors that you have been "practicing" for years. The good thing about the concept of drift is that we slip back to our old ways, and not suddenly. If we stay alert, we can catch drift early, reevaluate our motivational levels, and get back on track using the behavioral skills we have learned. The risk of drift will always be there, but the longer you stick with your new behaviors by using the SMART skills, the more motivated you will be, the stronger your habits will become, and the less impact the drift will have.

> Bill: "These basic principles and the SMART skills just don't apply to me. My problems are far more complicated."

Bill is a 45-year-old successful businessman, with a solid marriage and two small children. Throughout his early adult life, Bill was a dedicated athlete. He ran every day, lifted weights, ate a healthy diet, and focused a lot of attention on staying fit. Bill played football in college, but a serious knee injury during his senior year ended his athletic career.

Following his knee injury, Bill's lifestyle and conscientious health habits gradually changed. Following his marriage, he tried to stay fit by going to the gym. This seemed to work for a few years, but Bill began to slack off doing his regular exercise routine when he started managing a large car dealership. At the same time, his healthy diet began to deteriorate. Slowly, over the course of 15 years, Bill went from being a physically fit, college athlete to a 45-year-old, obese man.

Bill went to his doctor for a physical and found out he has high cholesterol, borderline hypertension, and is in the beginning stage of Type 2 diabetes. He has developed mild degenerative arthritis in his knee—the one with the old injury. Bill told us:

"I'm falling apart. I'm 45 years old, in terrible shape, and I'm going downhill fast. I have to change everything. I need to eat differently, exercise regularly, start taking medication, and reduce the stress in my life. How the heck am I going to do all this? It's just too much to handle if I expect to keep working and take care of my family. I understand the principles in the book, and I know the SMART skills, but my problems are more complicated. I need to make a lot of lifestyle changes—changes that involve every aspect of my life. I need more help than your basic principles and those simple behavior skills. My problems are too complicated."

Obviously, Bill had reached his limit both physically and emotionally. His body was telling him he could no longer keep up the same pace without some help. We talked about his need to change his health habits in the same way that you need to care for your car. Bill had been running his car at full speed for about 15 years without changing the oil, maintaining the brakes, keeping the transmission levels full, or lubricating the chassis. Now things were starting to fall apart.

Bill could relate to the car analogy. He went along with it, telling us he felt as if he was headed to the junkyard. He further stated that he knew how to fix his "car," but he didn't have the time or the skills to "overhaul" it. Because of this, he wakes up each day hoping the "car" will start. We let Bill know that many people find themselves in the same situation. Feeling overwhelmed is a common reaction to needing more than one lifestyle change. Bill was on a psychological merry-go-round. He knew he needed to make some significant changes in his life, but he didn't know where to start. As a result, his thoughts of needing to change just went around and around in his head, but he never did anything about it. We asked Bill if he felt "stuck," and he replied, "One hundred percent stuck." Bill was immobilized with thoughts and feelings about the changes he needed to make. He had no way to put his "transmission" into drive.

Despite being clear about the need to make several changes in his lifestyle, Bill needed to be challenged about his level of motivation. Was it possible that making the changes would be more trouble than it was worth? Bill admitted that sometimes he felt changing his health behavior was too much trouble, relative to the benefits to be gained, but he also knew he wanted to be healthy for his wife and children. He wanted to feel better, and he could see how his health problems were affecting his job performance and relationships. Bill told us he was scared. He was afraid he would fail if he tried to change.

We asked Bill to think about something other than his health. We wanted him to talk about things he understood, such as business and sports. Every business venture needs a strategy, and every competitive sport needs a game plan. Bill agreed that a person who has never run a business probably shouldn't start a multibillion dollar company, and a person who has never played a sport can't compete at the professional level. This was the case for Bill in dealing with his health. Other than his desire to change his lifestyle, he had no real plan; yet, he wanted to attempt a level of change he probably couldn't handle.

If you were asked to help Bill tackle the behavior changes he wanted to make, what suggestions would you offer? How could he begin to make these changes?

_____

_____

_____

_____

Of course, Bill was capable of making all of the necessary behavior changes, but he was overwhelmed by thinking about them all at once. We emphasized the importance of taking things one step at a time. Bill needed to re-think his situation. He needed to make multiple changes: in his diet, exercise program, medications, and stress management, and he needed to stick with them for the rest of his life. These were Bill's ultimate goals, but we asked him to focus on one thing he could do immediately that would move him along the path to better health.

Bill told us he could start a diet or exercise program, but that it seemed to be a huge and overwhelming task. And, he believed it would never work. Because each of the changes he needed to make seemed so big, Bill needed to scale way back. He needed to start with small, achievable goals that he was confident he could meet. We asked him to forget his exercise program for a minute and focus instead on what other behaviors he could do this week that would help him move toward his goals of better overall health.

It was as if a light bulb had been turned on in his head. "I could start doing the rehabilitation exercises for my knee," he said. "Maybe I could talk with my wife about what I should be eating to lose some of this weight. I know I need to take my medications. Let's see. What else?"

Bill was on a roll but, once again, he was trying to take on more changes than he could reasonably handle. Our recommendation was to begin with some knee exercises this week, add some simple changes in his eating habits next week, and consider the addition of some aerobic exercises to his routine in the third week. By a thoughtful and step-wise approach, Bill could ultimately have success, but Bill had to have clear goals and ones that he was sure he could achieve. This would allow him to be on his way to success.

However, Bill was stuck in a psychological "rut," and understandably feeling overwhelmed because of the need to make multiple lifestyle changes. He knew what he needed to do, and he wanted to make the needed changes, but he just couldn't get started. This happened because he was focused on the ultimate goals he was trying to achieve (weight loss, regular exercise, reduced stress, and medication compliance) without breaking them down into manageable behaviors. Bill needed to start small by using the SMART skills to do his knee exercises, make some small changes in his diet, and begin a structured medication regimen.

Bill didn't need to accomplish everything immediately. He didn't need to do it all; he just had to start doing something. Achievable goals and small initial behavioral changes were exactly what Bill needed to get the ball rolling.

Mike: "This is just common sense. What's the big deal about SMART skills?"

Mike is 57 years old. He's married, has two children, and works as an account executive for an advertising company. His son is beginning his junior year of college and his daughter just finished her freshman year. Now that his children are out of the house, he's decided it's time to get back in shape.

Mike has been relatively active throughout his life, but he's let his exercise habits slip and hasn't exercised consistently in about 10 years. An appendectomy, some prostate problems, and a busy lifestyle have left him about 15 pounds overweight. For the past few months, he hasn't been getting any physical activity that could be considered as exercise. Mike's wife gave him an earlier version of this book because she's watched him struggle with trying to make lasting health lifestyle changes. She thinks his ideas about getting healthy are great, and he definitely talks a good line. She believes he is motivated to make some serious changes in his exercise and eating behavior. The problem is that Mike thinks this is all he needs: a little motivation and some common sense. In fact, after he read the book, he said, "What's the big deal? This is all common sense. I just need to get started." Determined to get in shape, Mike joined the local gym and started watching what he eats. For 3 weeks he worked out every day and followed a strict diet. He lost 5 pounds, but he is exhausted and frustrated. He's hungry all the time, his knees hurt, and he's about to call it quits. Mike said:

"This is ridiculous. I am working out like a madman, and I've only lost 5 pounds. I know these lifestyle changes are good for me, but I'm starting to feel like it's not worth it. It shouldn't be this difficult. I'm just about ready to give up. This is my pattern, isn't it?"

How would you respond to Mike if you were coaching him? Can you identify any problems with what he is doing?

_____

_____

_____

_____

You probably recognized that Mike needs to revisit his goal in order to make sure it's clear, specific, and achievable. Helping him set a goal is a great place to start. Mike responded to our question about goals by indicating that he wants to lose 15 pounds and keep it off forever. He also wants to be in better overall physical shape.

Mike told us he anticipated it would take approximately a month to lose 15 pounds, but that he was hoping to lose the extra weight in less than 4 weeks by pushing himself to the limit. He thought he could be in good physical shape by then, too.

Mike's plan seemed in need of a reality check. It had taken quite a bit of time for him to get "out of shape"— about 10 years. How realistic was it to think he could get back into shape in less than 1 month? Was this an achievable goal? Was it clear and specific? Is it observable?

As much as he wanted this experience to be over quickly, Mike had set the bar too high. He wasn't focused on observable behavior that could help him reach his goals to get more physical activity and change his eating habits. Because Mike didn't set a behavior goal that was specific—one that he was sure he could achieve—his chances of success were slim from the beginning.

Mike was adamant about his motivation and persistence. "I'm giving it everything I have. I want this to happen, and I know that I'll get there if I just push myself."

This is where many people (especially men, for some reason) get it wrong. It's great to want to lose 15 pounds and get back in shape, but pushing too hard won't make the process go faster; instead, it will likely make you want to quit. Moreover, it's essential that Mike establishes realistic and reachable goals. If he doesn't, no matter how much motivation he has, he will run the risk of driving himself physically and mentally into the ground.

Mike honestly thought that losing 15 pounds was a good goal. At this point in our conversation, he appeared confused and asked us whether his goal might be unreasonable. Losing 15 pounds was not our concern, but Mike's unrealistic time frame and the fact that he wasn't tracking an observable behavior, such as changing his food choices, portions, or calories, could set him up for disappointment. Goals that can't be reached result in feelings of failure, and feelings of failure will reduce the chances of success in making positive lifestyle changes. Mike needed to break his goals into smaller, daily behaviors that were observable, measurable, and achievable.

We asked Mike to consider several questions about his behavioral targets, hoping that his answers would help him understand the importance of setting clear, specific, and achievable goals. How many days of the week was he going to exercise? For how long was he going to exercise? What specific activity was he planning to do? Where would he do the activity? What was he going to eat at each meal and where was he going to eat it? How many calories was he going to have daily? Was he going to follow a diet plan for every meal?

Mike immediately recognized that being specific would force him to look closely at what he was doing. By making his goals detailed, he could see them become measurable and more realistic. Finally, by having small daily goals instead of one big one, he could make the larger task much more manageable. In this way, short-term behavior goals could help Mike meet his long-term goals.

After his coaching sessions, Mike understood it was no surprise that he was tired, hungry, and frustrated. He decided that if he could focus on getting to the gym 4–5 days a week instead of 7, his behavior change strategy would be much more achievable. Mike finally had uttered the magic word, "achievable." This kind of "common sense" will get Mike where he wants to go.

What other advice would you give Mike to help him be successful with changes in his exercise and eating behaviors?

_____

_____

_____

_____

Hopefully, you advised him to add the remaining SMART skills into his plan. Monitoring, arranging his environment to help him be successful and make the target behaviors easy to do, recruiting support, and treating himself for meeting his goals will greatly increase his chances of getting into shape and losing 15 pounds. In fact, he will be successful if he follows all of these guidelines.

Finally, Mike is right that the SMART skills are common sense. It's not as if people haven't heard them before. Behavioral skills to help people change have been around for years, and they are simple and straightforward. However, thinking of the SMART skills only as "common sense" diminishes their power and discounts their potency. Mike is a great example of dismissing something that "everyone knows," thinking that it doesn't apply to him and struggling with lifestyle changes as a result. Putting common sense into action is the key, and it starts with knowing how to set a realistic goal and using the other SMART skills to set up your success.

> Donna: "I understand the formula and the SMART skills. I want to be healthy. I just need some motivation to exercise."

Donna is 40 years old and just beginning to feel the physical effects of getting a little older. She works full-time as a medical assistant for a busy primary care practice. She is a single mother of a 12-year-old son, and says that he is her top priority. Between his needs, her career, and a long commute to the office, Donna hasn't been able to fit exercise into her daily routine. She knows exercise is important to her overall health; she wants to be healthy, and she understands that exercise will help her feel better and keep her weight in check. Donna says her problem is a lack of motivation.

If you were coaching Donna and advising her as to what to do about her problem, what would you say? What would you recommend as the next step?

_____

_____

_____

_____

You may have noted that Donna does have some motivation. She stated that she wants to be healthy, and she recognizes the benefits of exercising. How could she take advantage of this available internal motivation? Does she need to examine her personal reasons for wanting to be healthier? Perhaps you advised Donna to get started on some type of activity program, even if it was a small beginning. If you suggested that the motivation she currently expressed is enough to get started—great! If Donna can leverage even a small amount of motivation to begin a behavior change program, she may discover that her motivation to continue will increase as she progresses toward her goal.

Donna didn't buy into the strategy of using what motivation she already has to get started. She still didn't understand how she could find the time to exercise, given her commitments and responsibilities. How could she possibly fit one more thing into her schedule? She described feeling defeated before even starting an exercise plan: "Where will I find the motivation to do this—I have to get more motivated." Donna spoke as if motivation was something she could buy off the shelf or find on the Internet. She thought if she just had enough motivation, she would succeed. Now, if she could only locate it.

We thought maybe we could help Donna locate some motivation and we knew the key was to help her find it within. Upon questioning her a bit more about her motivation with regard to exercise and the benefits she might experience, she described several more advantages: "I can lose weight, feel better, look better, be healthier, fit into my clothes, feel better about myself, and feel like I have some control over my life." This was a long list of benefits. We also asked Donna how important it was to her that she starts an exercise routine. She said, "Important."

When asked to put a number to her level of motivation, Donna rated her motivation to exercise at four on a ten-point scale. This number was relatively low, but clearly she has some internal level of desire to change her exercise habits. She was surprised when we told her that this level of motivation was adequate to get started.

How would you suggest Donna move forward, given that her motivation is enough to initiate a change in her behavior?

_____

_____

_____

_____

If you recommended that Donna begin with setting a clear goal for exercise, one she is certain she can achieve, you have provided excellent advice. Did you suggest that she start small? Because Donna is not exercising at all, anything she does will be a big improvement. The point is to use the little bit of motivation that she has to start doing something. Starting small will increase her chances of success, and the experience of success will bring about more confidence and motivation. Remember, motivation is self-perpetuating, and a small amount is enough to get Donna started. Of course, Donna also needs to use the remainder of the SMART skills to ensure long-term success. She knows all of the SMART skills and can recite them without difficulty.

What would you suggest to Donna if she needed any help with the SMART skills? What does she need to do to monitor her progress? How would you recommend that Donna arrange her world for success, recruit a support team, and treat herself?

_____

_____

_____

_____

Achieving success is simply a matter of putting the SMART skills into play. Donna had enough motivation to get going with a behavior change plan. She didn't have to do a lot of exercise; she just needed to do some. Even a small amount of activity—such as walking for 30 minutes, 3 days a week—was a big improvement from nothing, and Donna finally began to experience the benefits she expected from getting more physical activity.

12

More Action Tips

Get a Grip on Stress

We all experience stress at one time or another. What can you do when the pressures of life become too much? Stress has a way of building up to the point that you feel overwhelmed. The trick to managing it is to have a game plan. Try these suggestions:

➢ Make a list of the stressful situations in your life. Put a checkmark next to the ones you can change. Cross out the ones you can't. This will help you focus on what you can do versus what you can't.

➢ Don't let stressful thoughts grow bigger than the situation warrants. Take a look at the situations on your list. Can you think differently about some of them so they feel less stressful?

➢ Pay attention to your stress levels during the day. Every hour or so, take a minute to breathe deeply and collect your thoughts.

➢ Eat healthy, exercise regularly, and get enough rest. As hard as this seems, it will make you feel better and help you cope more effectively.

Plan ahead and take control when life gets crazy.

Help Your Children Lead More Active Lifestyles

With cable television, video games, phones, and the Internet, it's no wonder many children don't get enough exercise. Here is how you can help them become more physically active:

JOSHUA KLAPOW, SHERI PRUITT

- Ask them to list specific activities they can do for a set amount of time. Maybe it's kicking a soccer ball for 15 minutes, shooting baskets, or playing on a swing set.
- Use a calendar to help them keep track of how much exercise they get each day.
- Establish new routines, such as having them exercise before they watch television. They may resist at first, but they'll come around because exercising will make them feel good.
- Just as you reward your kids for good grades, reward them for sticking with their new activity habits.

H children. These tips will help you establish more active routines for them. And who knows—you may become more active as well.

Beating Road Rage

We've all heard about road rage and the deadly consequences of letting our emotions spin out of control. With our busy schedules and more of us on the road, it's easy for a little frustration to turn into full-blown road rage. Keeping your emotions in check is the key. Try these helpful tips:

- Focus on your breathing while driving, and make sure it's slow and steady. The more regulated your breathing, the more relaxed you'll feel.
- Loosen your grip on the steering wheel and drop your shoulders to help reduce muscle tension.
- Use music to regulate your mood. Listening to slow-paced relaxing music will reduce tension without your even trying.
- Set realistic time expectations—if you're in a hurry and late, you are almost guaranteed to be tense. Allow enough time to get where you're going.

Driving can be a frustrating experience, but it doesn't need to be a deadly one. Stay in control of your emotions and you'll be safer on the road.

Heart-Healthy Actions

Cardiovascular disease is the nation's number one killer. If you want to reduce your chances of heart disease here's what to do:

➢ Maintain a healthy weight using the concepts in this book to help your motivation level.
➢ Manage your blood pressure and cholesterol. Get them checked often. Sometimes your local pharmacy will do this for free or at a low cost.
➢ Reduce salt intake if you have high blood pressure; don't use it in cooking or add it at the table.
➢ Exercise.
➢ Don't smoke. Quit immediately if you do!
➢ Lower your stress levels when necessary. Take 10–15 minutes to relax your mind and body by using, for example, deep breathing or yoga exercises, listening to soothing music, taking a hot bath or shower, or removing yourself from a stressful situation by taking a walk.

Will doing these things today prevent heart disease? No, not in one day, but it is a start, and sometimes that's all you need.

Dealing with Holiday Stress

The holidays are supposed to be a time of joy and bliss, but for many people the preparations and obligations lead to added stress. Here are some tips to help you keep your holiday stress in check:

➢ Be realistic about the holidays. They don't need to be perfect to be joyous. Remind yourself that there will be good times and bad times.
➢ Remember that it's okay to feel stressed, sad, and angry during the holidays. Feeling bad doesn't mean the holidays are ruined.
➢ Slow down and prioritize your activities. You can't attend every party, buy every gift, cook every meal, and visit every relative. Write down everything you plan to do during

the holidays, and then read the list out loud. Is it a reasonable list? If not, start crossing things off.

➤ Pay attention to your health. Get plenty of sleep, try to eat right, manage your alcohol intake, and exercise when you can. Your holiday won't be joyous if you are sick or overstressed.

We all want the holidays to be a happy time. By having realistic expectations and not overextending, you will keep your stress levels in check and increase your enjoyment.

Managing the Holiday Blues

The holidays are a time of joy for most people. However, holiday time can also mean a bout of the "blues." Here are some tips that should help:

➤ Set realistic expectations for the holidays. As special as they are, they will not erase all of your past problems.

➤ Create new traditions if trying to re-create the old ones makes you sad.

➤ Remember that it's okay not to feel festive all of the time. If you are feeling down, just let others know.

➤ Take some time for yourself. Plan activities that you enjoy, and spend time with family or close friends.

➤ Be sure to get plenty of sleep, eat healthy meals, stay active, and limit your intake of alcohol.

What if someone you love has the blues?

➤ Try to involve that person in holiday activities, but don't be forceful.

➤ Be a good listener. Remember that the holidays can be a tough time for some people, and letting them talk about it may be all they need.

The good news is that, for most people, holiday blues are temporary. However, for some people, the holidays can bring on the more serious condition of clinical depression. If you or someone you know doesn't shake the blues after a few weeks, it's time to talk with your doctor or a mental health professional.

Holiday Spending

For many people holiday shopping results in heavy debt. Shopping is a behavior that often spins out of control. Here are some tips that will help you better manage your spending:

➤ Make a list of the people you are going to shop for and write down the total amount that you are going to spend on each of them.

➤ Take cash when you go shopping and leave the credit cards at home. Also, make sure you give yourself enough time to shop so that you won't be pressured into making last-minute impulse purchases. While you are shopping, write down every purchase and the price next to each person's name on your list.

➤ Make yourself accountable by letting one other person know how much you have budgeted. Being accountable to someone else will help you maintain control.

➤ Set aside some funds as an incentive for staying within your budget. You can purchase something for yourself or give it to charity.

With a bit of planning you can reduce the stress of overspending and really enjoy the holiday shopping experience.

Talking about Emotional Problems

Everyone feels sad or anxious at one time or another. But what do you do when those feelings start getting the best of you? You may feel awkward when talking with your doctor, but emotional problems are just as serious and treatable as physical problems. To make it easier, talk with your doctor about your emotional symptoms just as you would about physical symptoms. Tell your doctor when the symptoms started, how often they occur, and how the symptoms are impacting your daily life.

Make sure you discuss and understand your treatment options. This might mean psychotherapy, medication, or a follow-up visit. This strategy will make the conversation easier, but the most important action you can take is to follow through with treatment. If left untreated, emotional symptoms can get much worse.

Being a Caregiver

Nearly 21 percent of Americans provide care for a chronically ill or disabled loved one over the age of 18. But caregiving can take a toll on the mind and body. Taking care of your own health is one of the most important things you can do. If you become ill, who will do the caregiving? Here are some simple ways to make sure you care for yourself:

➢ Stay healthy. Make sure you eat well, get enough sleep, and exercise each day.
➢ Keep a journal of your thoughts and feelings. It's a great release for your emotions.
➢ Do one activity that you enjoy every day.
➢ Set aside time to be with others for an evening out or having friends over to visit.
➢ Ask for help from a friend, family member, or professional organization. You don't have to do this alone.

You may feel guilty about focusing on yourself, but these efforts will help you feel better and give you the strength you need to be the best caregiver possible.

13

You CAN Do This

There you have it! As we promised at the beginning of this book, you now have everything you need to make any lifestyle change you desire. Stop for just a moment and think about this, because it's important. You now have a foundation for living a healthier life and creating long-term habits. You may choose not to use it, but whenever you want to change a health-related behavior you have the basic principles and skills you need. Think about all of the health-related behaviors that you could improve using the ideas in this book. Having The What, The Want, and SMART skills to accomplish The How can empower you to change your life. More importantly, when you make changes in your lifestyle, you will be able to stick with it.

Life gets in the way of our intentions and a plan, so having a strategy to stay on course is critical. You will drift from your healthy behaviors from time to time, and sometimes you will feel your motivation slipping, but you can remind yourself that when it's time to get back on track you have everything you need. Living SMART is not about being perfect, it's about making the right choices and engaging in the right behaviors more days than not. Remember the "What Ifs," your drift partner, and the three-day rule. If you skip a workout or stray from your eating plan, you have made one "bad" choice and engaged in one "bad" behavior, but immediately you can use the SMART skills to get moving again in a positive direction. Use the SMART skills and you'll always be on track with your lifestyle goals. We're confident you will do a great job. Congratulations, you are on your way to living a healthier life.

Joshua C. Klapow, Ph.D.
Sheri D. Pruitt, Ph.D.

Appendix A
Charts for Change

This section includes some reminders, copies of some of the charts in the book, as well as additional interactive exercises to help you reach your lifestyle goals. These can be photocopied to make sure you have enough as you go along.

The Chart **The What, The Want, and The How**
My health behavior is: _____(be specific) I will practice my behavior_____days per week. My short-term goal is _____. My long-term goal is_____. I will give myself _____(treat) on the following schedule: _____(how often). In addition to giving myself _____, when I complete _____ (number of days, weeks, or months), I will give myself a bonus treat of _____.

SUN	MON	TUE	WED	THU	FRI	SAT

Interactive Exercises to Increase Your Motivation

These fast and easy exercises will help you increase your motivation levels by tapping into what's already inside you. They can be done any time you feel your motivation slipping. Doing them from time to time will help you remember your reasons for changing your lifestyle.

Forecasting Your Future. What if you aren't sure you are motivated enough to make a change? Stop for a moment and think about what is really important to you. If you don't change your health habits, will you still be here 5 years from now? Will you be able to work, go on vacation, be with your family, and enjoy your life? Will you be able to do the things that make your life worth living? Your future and your ability to function in that future are determined in large part by what you do every day. Ask yourself these questions and write down your answers:

➢ What concerns do you have about your health?

_____.

➢ What things are you currently doing to be healthier?

_____.

➢ If you could make some improvements in your health, how would you feel?

_____.

➢ What else would be different about you?

_____.

➢ What would be better for your loved ones if you made health improvements?

_____.

➢ What behavior have you been able to successfully change in the past?

_____.

➢ When do you plan to get started?

_____.

By taking the time to answer these questions, most of you will be reminded of why you set out to make changes in your lifestyle in the first place. Simple as it seems, this little reminder about what is important to you and your reasons for wanting to change can really boost your level of motivation. So, if you ever find your motivation slipping, repeat this exercise.

Is Making This Change Important? How important is making a specific behavior change? Use the scales below to rate how important it is for you to make the behavioral change you're considering and how confident you are that you will succeed.

1. How important is it that I make the change?

    1   2   3   4   5   6   7   8   9   10

    Not important   Extremely important

2. What would make this behavioral change more important?

    _____

    _____.

3. Am I confident I can make the change?

    1   2   3   4   5   6   7   8   9   10

    Not confident at all   Extremely confident

4. What would make you more confident?

    _____

    _____.

By answering these questions, you have likely discovered a number of reasons for changing an unhealthy behavior. You've probably realized that your emotions play a significant role in your decision to make the change. Thinking about changing a behavior can bring up a variety of emotions, including anger, fear of failure, and anxiety. While change can be difficult and stressful, consider the consequences of not changing. What are you doing today to become the healthy person you envision yourself being in the future? What benefits do you expect from making a healthy change? How long can you afford to wait before doing things differently to improve your health?

Tips for Dealing with Negative Thoughts. You can be sailing along and then—all of a sudden—it happens. You experience some small setback in your diet, exercise program, or management of your blood pressure, and then the flood of negative thoughts comes. This type of thinking will dampen your motivation, but it doesn't have to mean the end of your success. Here is a simple strategy for managing negative thoughts:

1. Catch yourself when you experience a negative thought. Negative thoughts most often occur following a slip-up. Take a minute to write down your answers to the following questions: What's going through my mind? What am I saying to myself? What are my thoughts? Maybe they are something like: "I have no self-control" or "I'm not disciplined enough to do this."

2. Turn the negative thought into an action. Once you've caught the negative thought and written it down, repeat it out loud, but imagine someone else is saying it to you. Imagine, for example, that someone said: "You have no self-control" or "You're just not disciplined enough." By picturing someone else saying the words, you will be more likely to stick up for yourself. This takes us to the third step.

3. Defend yourself. Do you really lack self-control? Chances are this negative thought isn't 100 percent accurate. Think about the times when you have shown self-control, and write down as many examples as you can to prove that this negative thought is not true. Also, think about other explanations for why you slipped up this time.

This exercise won't keep you from having negative thoughts, and it won't prevent occasional slip-ups. It will, however, keep one slip-up and one negative thought from taking over and ruining your efforts. By catching your negative thoughts and managing them, you will be able to keep your focus on what is important to you and chose behaviors in line with your goals.

SMART Skills

Using the SMART skills can be the difference between people who make lifestyle changes and stick with them, and people who try but don't succeed. Here are two examples using the common health behaviors of exercise and eating.

Exercise: The five skills you need to use if you want to become more physically active are:

Set a clear, achievable goal.

Be sure your exercise goal is specific and that it can be measured. For example, "I will walk 30 minutes, 3 days a week" is a clear, specific, and measurable goal. The more specific you can be with your goal, the better it is for your success. Start small—choose a goal you can accomplish and one that will boost your confidence, and then build on your success.

Monitor your progress.

Track your progress using a simple calendar so that you have a visible "report card" of your exercise behavior changes over time. Put an "x" on each day that you meet your goal. If you're not accomplishing what you planned, you can check the calendar for patterns and adjust your behavior or modify your goal. Start by ensuring that your goal is achievable—if you're not meeting it, maybe it needs to be more achievable. Use The Chart in Chapter 6 to keep track of your progress; for example, to record the number of minutes (in 5-minute increments) that you exercise each day. Remember, monitoring behavior changes behavior. Watch your progress and be proud of yourself!

Arrange your world for success.

Create an environment that makes it easy to do the right thing. Arrange your surroundings to make it easy to do your target behavior. If you are working on exercise, put your gym bag in your car so you have everything you need for a workout. Post a picture of a walker or a runner above your desk to remind you what you're working toward. Put your monitoring form in a place you will see every day, such as the refrigerator door or the bathroom mirror. Schedule an exercise session in your calendar and set an alarm on your phone.

Recruit a support team.

Enlist the help of others. Let the people who want to see you succeed know what you're trying to achieve. Consider your family, friends, and work colleagues as your potential support team. Ask them to support your efforts in meeting your activity goals, and to join you in celebrating your success. Let them know exactly how they can help you meet your exercise goals. Your supporters will be happy to help you and let you know you're doing a great job!

JOSHUA KLAPOW, SHERI PRUITT

Treat yourself.

Reward yourself every time you do the behavior you have targeted. Treat yourself after every walk, every gym session, or every time you meet your activity goals. Do all you can to pair good feelings, like success and accomplishment, with exercise. Select a "treat" that is important to you, readily available, and not costly. An internal celebration, 10 minutes of alone time, or a chat with your exercise partner are some good examples of treats. Treats are especially important when you are starting a new exercise behavior— treat yourself every time. You can phase them out as the new exercise behavior becomes more automatic and habitual.

Eating Behaviors: If you want to change your eating habits, the same five skills look like this:

Set a clear, achievable goal.

Be sure your eating goal is specific and is something you can measure. For example, "I will eat three servings of fruits and vegetables a day" is an example of a clear, specific, and measurable goal. Start small—choose a goal you can accomplish, which builds your confidence, and then build upon your success.

Monitor your progress.

Keep track of what you eat. You can use a simple calendar to monitor your eating behavior over time. Put an "x" on each day that you meet your goal. Look for patterns and make adjustments if you're not accomplishing what you planned. Consider modifying your goal if you can't accomplish it. Watch your progress and feel proud! Remember, monitoring behavior changes behavior.

Arrange your world for success.

Arrange your environment to help you be successful with your eating goals. Make it easy for you to eat the foods on your plan. Put your monitoring form in a place you see every day, such as the refrigerator door or your bathroom mirror. Keep healthy foods available and don't bring the foods you don't want to eat into your surroundings (your car, office, and home). It is that simple. You will eat what is available to you.

Recruit a support team.

Enlist the help of others. Let those who want to see you succeed know what you're trying to achieve and exactly how they can support you. Consider your family, friends, and work

116

colleagues as your potential support team. Ask them to support your efforts in meeting your eating goals and to join you in celebrating your success. Supporters will be happy to encourage you and let you know you're doing a great job!

Treat yourself.

Reward yourself every time you do the eating behavior you have targeted. Select a "treat" that is important to you, readily available, and not costly. Telling yourself, "Great job!" works well. A special low-calorie beverage, a few minutes of alone time, or imagining yourself getting another trophy are some good examples of treats. The idea is to pair strong, positive feelings with eating healthy foods. Rewarding yourself is especially important in the beginning, when you are starting a new eating behavior. Treat yourself every time to connect good feelings of success and accomplishment with healthy eating.

You can apply this same set of skills to any health behavior you want to change—or any behavior at all, for that matter.

If You Need More Help with SMART Skills and Behavioral Drift

Setting an Exercise Goal. Did you know that even a small amount of exercise can improve your health and fitness? Regular exercise can reduce your risk of a number of health problems, including chronic pain, diabetes, and stress. Your overall well-being can improve significantly after making even small lifestyle changes in the area of exercise.

People who are successful at starting new exercise habits begin with clear, achievable goals: specific, measurable, and observable. The more specific your goal, the more likely you are to achieve it. Here are some examples of good and not so good goals for exercising:

"Exercise More" is a nice idea, but not specific enough to be a good goal.

"Walk 5 miles a day" is specific and measurable, but probably not realistic if you aren't already walking regularly.

"Walk 30 minutes 7 days a week at lunchtime" is more attainable, but what if you have an extra busy day or the weather is sometimes bad at noon?

"Walk 30 minutes, 5 days a week" is specific, measurable, and observable, and it is something you can likely achieve and can boost your confidence about exercising.

Here are some questions to ask yourself in order to help you set a behavioral goal for exercise.

1. This week, what do you specifically want to achieve?

    Which activity do you want to do?

    >   Walking   Running   Biking   Swimming   Other_____

    - How much time do you want to spend exercising on the days that you exercise?

        >   5 minutes   10 minutes   15 minutes   20 minutes   Half Hour

    - How many days a week do you want to exercise?

        >   1 day   2 days   3 days   4 days   5 days   6 days   7 days

2. Is your exercise goal something you can see and measure?

    A good goal can be measured and monitored so that you will know if you met it.

    - How will I keep track of my exercise this week?

        >   chart   diary   calendar   phone   Other_____

3. Is your goal for the week realistic?

    A good goal is something you are likely to achieve. Make sure you have the time to do it and everything you need to achieve it. Many people have busy days, and you may need to plan carefully to fit exercise into your schedule. Setting an exercise goal that you can't achieve sets you up for feelings of failure and disappointment. Don't do this. It is self-defeating and unnecessary.

My activity goal for this week is:

The activity: _____

The number of days per week: _____

The number of minutes per day: _____

How confident am I that I can I meet this goal? _____

Setting an Eating Goal. Whether you want to eat more fruits and vegetables, eat fewer calories, reduce your portion size, or cut out sweets, the way you set your goal is critical for your success. You get to determine what it is, so don't set a goal that is too difficult to accomplish.

People who are successful at starting new eating habits begin with clear, achievable goals. Your goal should be specific, something that can be measured or counted, and something that can be seen if another person was watching you. Remember, the more specific you can be in setting your eating goal, the better your chances of success. Here are some examples of good and not so good goals for changing eating habits:

"I want to eat a healthier diet" is a nice idea, but not specific enough to be a good goal.

"I want to eat five servings of fruits and vegetables every day" is specific and measurable, but probably not realistic if you haven't been eating fruits and vegetables at all.

"I want to eat two servings of fruits and vegetables every day at lunchtime" is more attainable, but what if you have an extra busy day and cannot find healthy food?

"I want to eat two servings of fruits and vegetables, 3 days a week" is specific, measurable, and observable, and it is something you can likely achieve.

Here are some questions to ask yourself that will help you set a behavioral goal about eating.

1.   This week, what do you specifically want to achieve?

   •   Which eating habit do you want to change?

       more fruits/   fewer   reduce fast   limit sweets   Other_____
       vegetables   calories   food

   •   How many days per week do you want to target for changing your eating habits?

       2 days   3 days   5 days   7 days   Other_____

2.   Is your eating goal something you can see and measure?

   A good goal includes a behavior that can be measured or counted, and monitored so you will be able to track your progress.

   •   How will I keep track of my eating behavior this week?

       monitoring chart   food diary   calendar   phone app   Other_____

3.   Is your goal realistic for this week?

   A good goal is something you are quite confident you can achieve. Make sure that you have everything you need to meet the goal you've set with regard to eating behaviors. Have the foods you want to eat available. We all have busy days and unexpected interruptions. Think about back-up plans when things change (the What-Ifs). You will need to plan carefully to fit your new eating habits into your schedule.

My eating goal for this week is: _____
The number of days per week I will work on my eating habits:_____
How confident am I that I can I meet this goal? _____

Monitor Your Progress

Self-Monitoring Form for Exercise. Use a chart like the one below to keep track of your progress as you begin your new exercise routine. A calendar can serve the same purpose. Remember that monitoring is a very powerful SMART skill. This chart is marked for someone who has a goal of walking 10 minutes per day the first week, 15 minutes per day the second week, and 20 minutes per day the third week.

Minutes	M	T	W	Th	F	S	S	M	T	W	Th	F	S	S	M	T	W	Th	F	S	S
70																					
65																					
60																					
55																					
50																					
45																					
40																					
35																					
30																					
25																					
20																					
15																					
10																					
5																					

Determine your activity goal for the first few weeks. It's a good idea to identify this in some way on your monitoring form. Next, place a check mark in the boxes representing the number of minutes that you exercise each day. In the example above, if you started a walking program on Monday, and you walked 10 minutes, you could put a check mark in the 5-minute box and one in the 10-minute box. If you fulfill your goal, all of the colored boxes will have a check at the end of the week.

You could also keep track of your total minutes of exercise. Simply record the number of minutes in the same place every day (on your calendar or on your phone app) and watch your progress.

Self-Monitoring Form for Eating. Use a chart like this one to keep track of your progress as you begin your new eating habits. A calendar can serve the same purpose. Remember to record each time you do your target behavior. You can keep track of calories, or use a simple check mark for breakfast, lunch, or dinner that meets your eating goal. Monitoring is a very powerful SMART skill. Monitoring what you eat can change your behavior.

Week 1							Week 2							Week 3							Week 4						
M	T	W	T	F	S	S	M	T	W	T	F	S	S	M	T	W	T	F	S	S	M	T	W	T	F	S	S

Determine your eating goal for the first two weeks. It's a good idea to identify this in some way on your monitoring form. Next, place a check mark in the boxes each day that you met your goal. For example, if you start a new eating habit on Monday, and you took a low-calorie, healthy lunch to work for five days, then you could check each box in the middle row for Monday, Tuesday, Wednesday, Thursday, and Friday.

You can make as many copies of this monitoring form as you need to keep track of the behavior over time, or you can create another form that works better for you—use whatever best allows you to keep track of your eating behavior. Monitoring your behavior is what matters. Use a format that works for you.

Arrange Your World for Success. Arranging your world for success is all about taking control of your environment in small but powerful ways. Making and sticking with changes will become easier and easier if you can arrange your surroundings to support the eating or exercise behaviors you are trying to change. Think of everything you can put in place to ensure you will do the target behavior. Your environment can "pull" behavior from you, so arrange it to "pull" your target behaviors. On the lines below, list the eating or exercise behavior that you want to change. Next, take the time to list the things you can do to set up the world around you to ensure your success.

Behavior I want to change: _____

Ways I can arrange my environment to support this change:

1. _____

2. _____

3. _____

4. _____

5. _____

Treat Yourself Checklist. Behaviors that are rewarded are more likely to be repeated. This is a well-known fact of human behavior that you can use to your advantage. Give yourself a "treat" each time you perform an activity or behavior that you want to continue. Treats can be short-term and long-term. Think about them in advance and don't leave to chance how you will treat yourself. Short-term rewards after exercising might include 10 minutes of alone time, watching the sunset at the end of your walk, or telling yourself "great job."

Long-term rewards can include new walking shoes or work-out clothes that you give yourself only after you have accumulated a pre-determined number of days of success with the target behavior. For example, you can give yourself a point every day you meet your exercise goal and when you accumulate 20 points you can buy something as a special treat.

Treats need to be meaningful to you! They need to be immediate! Plan them in advance so that you know what you're working toward. Treat yourself with something every time and choose in advance what will reward your target behavior. Celebrate your success!

Make a list of short-term rewards:

1. _____

2. _____

3. _____

4. _____

5. _____

Make a list of long-term rewards:

1. _____

2. _____

3. _____

4. _____

5. _____

I will give myself_____ as a reward for each time I do _____ (the target behavior).

I can treat myself by saying to myself _____ because internal rewards are powerful.

If I treat myself with points (or stars) after each behavior, after I meet my exercise goals for one month (or accumulate 20 points), I will reward myself with a special, bonus treat of_____.

Getting Back on Track

"What If..." Exercise

This "What If..." list will help you target situations that are likely to lead to behavioral drift. You know yourself better than anyone and you know the things that take you off track. The details will be different for each lifestyle behavior, but the process and general topics are the same.

Here are some common examples of events that take people off track with lifestyle changes. Consider what you will do when a "What If" happens to you. For practice, come up with a plan for each of the situations listed below

> ➢ What if the weather is bad and I can't exercise outside?
> Even if the weather is bad, I will _____.

> ➢ What if we go out to dinner and they don't have the foods on my diet?
> Even if I can't get the foods on my diet, I will _____.

> ➢ What if we are traveling and I can't get to bed at a reasonable hour?
> Even if I can't get to bed, I will _____.

> ➢ What if I go to a bar and someone offers me a cigarette?
> Even if I am offered a cigarette, I will _____.

> ➢ What if my schedule changes and I can't do my relaxation exercises in the morning before work?
> Even if my schedule changes, I will _____.

> ➢ What if my motivation levels decrease?
> Even if my motivation decreases, I will _____.

> ➢ What if I am sick or injured, and unable to exercise, prepare certain meals, or take my scheduled medications?
> Even if I am sick or injured, I will _____.

> ➢ What if my supporters are no longer available?
> Even if my supporters are not available, I will _____.

List three or more "What If" scenarios that might affect *your* success in achieving your lifestyle goals and what you plan to do.

1. _____

2. _____

3. _____

4. _____

5. _____

These situations will not necessarily cause behavioral drift, but they are good warning signs and can start the process if not caught early. Therefore, the longer your list of events, the better you will be able to plan. If you can anticipate it, you can plan for it—and if you can plan for it, you can plan how to deal with it.

Three-Day Rule Pledge

Use the pledge below to help you stick with the three-day rule. Remember, the three-day rule is to help you get back on track as quickly as possible and to stay alert for behavioral drift. Copy it from this book, fill it out, and post it where you can see it regularly.

My Three-Day Rule Pledge. If I stop doing the behaviors I have set out to reach my goals for a period of three days, for ANY reason, I will sit down and answer the following questions in writing:

1. What happened to get me off track?

    _____.

2. Which SMART skill can I use to get started again immediately?

    _____.

3. Exactly when do I plan to get back on track?

    _____.

4. I will post the start-up date on the refrigerator or some other location that I can easily see.

Date: _____

Signature: _____

References

Fisher, J.D. and Fisher, W.A. (1992) Changing AIDS-Risk Behaviour. Psychological Bulletin, 111, 455-474. http://dx.doi.org/10.1037/0033-2909.111.3.455

Fisher J.D. and Fisher W.A. (2000) Theoretical Approaches to Individual-Level Change in HIV Risk Behavior. In: Peterson J.L., DiClemente R.J. (eds) Handbook of HIV Prevention. Aids Prevention and Mental Health. Springer, Boston, MA.

Fisher, W. A., Fisher, J. D. and Harman, J. (2003) The Information-Motivation-Behavioral Skills Model: A General Social Psychological Approach to Understanding and Promoting Health Behavior, in Social Psychological Foundations of Health and Illness (eds J. Suls and K. A. Wallston), Blackwell Publishing Ltd, Malden, MA, USA. doi: 10.1002/9780470753552.ch4;

Sun Ju Chang, Suyoung Choi, Se-An Kim, Misoon Song. (2014) Intervention Strategies Based on Information-Motivation-Behavioral Skills Model for Health Behavior Change: A Systematic Review, In Asian Nursing Research, Volume 8, Issue 3, Pages 172-181, ISSN 1976-1317, https://doi.org/10.1016/j.anr.2014.08.002. (http://www.sciencedirect.com/science/article/pii/S1976131714000504)

Mazzuca, S. A. (1982) Does patient education in chronic disease have therapeutic value?, In Journal of Chronic Diseases, Volume 35, Issue 7, 1982, Pages 521-529, ISSN 0021-9681, https://doi.org/10.1016/0021-9681(82)90071-6. (http://www.sciencedirect.com/science/article/pii/0021968182900716)

Miller, W.R. and Rollnick, S. (2013) Motivational Interviewing: Helping People Change. Guilford Press: New York.

Butryn, M. L., Phelan, S., Hill, J. O. and Wing, R. R. (2007) Consistent Self-monitoring of Weight: A Key Component of Successful Weight Loss Maintenance. Obesity, 15: 3091–3096. doi:10.1038/oby.2007.368

Skinner, B.F. (1953) Science and Human Behavior. The Free Press: New York.

Marlatt, G. A. and George, W. H. (1984) Relapse Prevention: Introduction and Overview of the Model. British Journal of Addiction, 79: 261–273. doi:10.1111/j.1360-0443.1984.tb00274.x

Institute of Medicine, Board on Health Sciences Policy, Committee on Sleep Medicine and Research. (2006) Sleep Disorders and Sleep Deprivation: An Unmet Public Health Problem.

Osterberg, L. and Blaschke, T. (2005) Adherence to Medication. N Engl J Med 2005; 353:487-497, 2005 DOI: 10.1056/NEJMra05010